Case Studies
in Insomnia

CRITICAL ISSUES IN PSYCHIATRY
An Educational Series for Residents and Clinicians
Series Editor: Sherwyn M. Woods, M.D., Ph.D.
University of Southern California School of Medicine
Los Angeles, California

Recent volumes in the series:

CASE STUDIES IN INSOMNIA
Edited by Peter J. Hauri, Ph.D.

CLINICAL DISORDERS OF MEMORY
Aman U. Khan, M.D.

CONTEMPORARY PERSPECTIVES ON PSYCHOTHERAPY WITH LESBIANS AND GAY MEN
Edited by Terry S. Stein, M.D., and Carol J. Cohen, M.D.

DECIPHERING MOTIVATION IN PSYCHOTHERAPY
David M. Allen, M.D.

DIAGNOSTIC AND LABORATORY TESTING IN PSYCHIATRY
Edited by Mark S. Gold, M.D., and A. L. C. Pottash, M.D.

DRUG AND ALCOHOL ABUSE: A Clinical Guide to Diagnosis and Treatment, Third Edition
Marc A. Schuckit, M.D.

EMERGENCY PSYCHIATRY: Concepts, Methods, and Practices
Edited by Ellen L. Bassuk, M.D., and Ann W. Birk, Ph.D.

ETHNIC PSYCHIATRY
Edited by Charles B. Wilkinson, M.D.

EVALUATION OF THE PSYCHIATRIC PATIENT: A Primer
Seymour L. Halleck, M.D.

NEUROPSYCHIATRIC FEATURES OF MEDICAL DISORDERS
James W. Jefferson, M.D., and John R. Marshall, M.D.

THE RACE AGAINST TIME: Psychotherapy and Psychoanalysis in the Second Half of Life
Edited by Robert A. Nemiroff, M.D., and Calvin A. Colarusso, M.D.

STATES OF MIND: Configurational Analysis of Individual Psychology, Second Edition
Mardi J. Horowitz, M.D.

A Continuation Order Plan is available for this series. A continuation order will bring delivery of each new volume immediately upon publication. Volumes are billed only upon actual shipment. For further information please contact the publisher.

Case Studies in Insomnia

Edited by
PETER J. HAURI, Ph. D.
Mayo Clinic
Rochester, Minnesota

With a Foreword by
WILLIAM C. DEMENT, M.D., Ph.D.

Plenum Medical Book Company • New York and London

Library of Congress Cataloging-in-Publication Data

Case studies in insomnia / edited by Peter J. Hauri ; with a foreword
by William C. Dement.
    p.   cm. -- (Critical issues in psychiatry)
  Includes bibliographical references and index.
  ISBN 0-306-43791-0
  1. Insomnia--Treatment--Case studies.   I. Hauri, Peter.
II. Series.
  [DNLM: 1. Behavior Therapy--methods. 2. Insomnia--psychology.
3. Insomnia--therapy. 4. Psychotherapy--methods.   WM 188 C337]
RC548.C37 1991
616.8'498--dc20
DNLM/DLC
for Library of Congress   91-20965
                                                           CIP

ISBN 0-306-43791-0

© 1991 Plenum Publishing Corporation
233 Spring Street, New York, N.Y. 10013

Plenum Medical Book Company is an imprint of Plenum Publishing Corporation

All rights reserved

No part of this book may be reproduced, stored in a retrieval system, or transmitted
in any form or by any means, electronic, mechanical, photocopying, microfilming,
recording, or otherwise, without written permission from the Publisher

Printed in the United States of America

Contributors

Richard P. Allen   Sleep Disorders Center, Johns Hopkins University School of Medicine, Baltimore, Maryland 21224

Richard R. Bootzin   Department of Psychology, University of Arizona, Tucson, Arizona 85721

Andrew J. Borson   Sleep Disorders Center, Crozer-Chester Medical Center, Chester, Pennsylvania 19013

William C. Dement   Sleep Disorders Center, Stanford University, Palo Alto, California 94305

Dana Epstein   Department of Psychology, University of Arizona, Tucson, Arizona 85721

Milton K. Erman   Sleep Disorders Center, Scripps Clinic and Research Foundation, La Jolla, California 92037

Judith Flaxman   Illinois School of Professional Psychology, Chicago, Illinois 60604

Paul B. Glovinsky   Department of Psychology, The City College of the City University of New York, New York, New York 10031 and Insomnia Treatment Center, New York, New York 10017

Peter J. Hauri   Sleep Disorders Center, Mayo Clinic, Rochester, Minnesota 55905

John H. Koewler   Sleep Disorders and Research Center, Deaconess Hospital, St. Louis, Missouri 63139

Patricia Lacks   Psychology Department, Washington University, St. Louis, Missouri 63130

Stuart J. Menn Sleep Disorders Center, Scripps Clinic and Research Foundation, La Jolla, California 92037

Merrill M. Mitler Sleep Disorders Center, Scripps Clinic and Research Foundation, La Jolla, California 92037

Sidney D. Nau Sleep Disorders and Research Center, Deaconess Hospital, St. Louis, Missouri 63139

Steven Poceta Sleep Disorders Center, Scripps Clinic and Research Foundation, La Jolla, California 92037

Russell Rosenberg Northside Hospital, Atlanta, Georgia 30342

Thomas Roth Sleep Disorders and Research Center, Henry Ford Hospital, Detroit, Michigan 48202

Arthur J. Spielman Department of Psychology, The City College of the City University of New York, New York, New York 10031 and Insomnia Treatment Center, New York, New York 10017

Neil Steinberg Clinical Sleep Services, Santa Rosa, California 95402

Edward J. Stepanski Sleep Disorders and Research Center, Henry Ford Hospital, Detroit, Michigan 48202

Michael M. Stevenson North Valley Sleep Disorders Center, Mission Hills, California 91345

James K. Walsh Sleep Disorders and Research Center, Deaconess Hospital, St. Louis, Missouri 63139

Marsha K. Weinstein North Valley Sleep Disorders Center, Mission Hills, California 91345

James W. Wood Department of Psychology, University of Arizona, Tucson, Arizona 85721

Vincent P. Zarcone, Jr. Palo Alto VA Medical Center, Palo Alto, California 94304 and Department of Psychiatry, Stanford University School of Medicine, Stanford, California 94304

Frank J. Zorick Sleep Disorders and Research Center, Henry Ford Hospital, Detroit, Michigan 48202

Foreword

If ever a book could be called timely, this is it. Sleep disorders medicine has made rapid advances in recent years. The field has attained growing respectability, with a textbook recently published, a congressionally mandated National Commission on Sleep Disorders Research, and a growing public awareness of the importance of sleep disorders. However, this rapid growth has made the discrepancy among certain components of the field all the more obvious. Thus, we find that patients who complain of insomnia are almost never in the majority of those seen in sleep disorders centers, in spite of the well-known fact that the prevalence of such individuals in our society is by far the largest.

Current articles on insomnia abound, but they tend to be facile recitations of diagnosis and impractical global recommendations for treatment, without providing the essential details. Indeed, the clinical professions really do not know what to do about insomnia. This is reflected in a number of observations I have made in the recent past. For example, the majority of individuals who complain of insomnia take alcohol, aspirin, over-the-counter medications, hot baths, and a host of other nostrums, but rarely seek a physician. In the unlikely event that a physician is consulted, he is likely to prescribe a sleep medication but without any particular consistency, or any clear instructions on its use.

For the most part, patients who have insomnia go to doctors for other reasons, and even in these cases, no interaction about the problem takes place. We have carried out studies of clinical practices where we find that only from 2 to 10 percent of patients may spontaneously present sleep complaints to their doctors, but when questioned following office visits, 40 to 60 percent of these patients reveal that they have sleep complaints. We have come to believe that doctors do not want to ask about sleep problems because they do not know what to do to alleviate them.

In dramatic contrast to the above statement, the authors of this book do know what to do, and they tell us in clear, precise detail. Hallelujah!

Editor Peter Hauri has pulled together the knowledge and expertise about insomnia and has made the council of these experts available to patients and their therapists. Furthermore, much of the clinical experience documented in this book can be available in sleep disorders centers.

Although some feel (quite rightly) that sleep disorders medicine has come of age, it cannot claim full maturity until clear guidelines for the effective diagnosis and treatment of insomnia are in place. Whether this comes about in terms of performing more effectively as a tertiary center or a consultative service offering expertise and advice to primary care physicians, or as a kind of cooperative effort, or whether or not the diagnosis and treatment can become so efficient that patients should go directly to their local sleep disorders center, one cannot tell. However, it is absolutely time to get moving. One could easily estimate, from reading this book, that at least 75 percent of all chronic insomnia patients can benefit. Formidable problems remain, but the path is clear, and success, if sleep disorders specialists are willing to make the effort and follow many of the principles outlined in this book, is almost guaranteed.

If the population of the earth is over five billion individuals, and if the various prevalence reports for serious chronic insomnia are reasonably accurate, perhaps a billion people have insomnia. What a sad thing for life to be suboptimal for so many people.

Peter J. Hauri has been dedicated to the problem of insomnia since his days with Allen Rechtschaffen at the University of Chicago, which resulted in a doctoral thesis in 1966. He received the prestigious Nathaniel Kleitman prize for 1989, awarded by the American Sleep Disorders Association. Among other things, he was commended for his consistent contributions to the problem of insomnia.

I was honored and pleased to be asked to write this foreword, particularly because I had a chance to read the book perhaps a year or so before I otherwise would have seen it. I can sincerely say that the authors have done a great service for sleep specialists and insomniacs the world over. It is quite true, as Peter J. Hauri says, that much of the good work on insomnia has not been published. It would be a challenge to bring the different approaches discussed in this book together in one central place, but that is a happy challenge, with the likelihood of a favorable outcome. In the Preface, Dr. Hauri also comments that he hopes the book will go "beyond a mere 'how-to-do-it' cookbook," but even "how to do it" is of inestimable value to us all, and just what we do not have currently. I cannot think of a better example where a huge need has been met so decisively.

William C. Dement, M.D., Ph.D.

Sleep Disorders Center
Stanford University
Palo Alto, California

Preface

There has been a quiet revolution in the treatment of insomnia. Twenty years ago, insomnia was seen either as a manifestation of depression and anxiety or as an annoying disorder to be extinguished with hypnotics. In the late 1960s, I once asked Dr. Jacobson, who developed the progressive relaxation technique, if he ever used it to treat insomnia. He seemed annoyed and said, in essence, that insomniacs were a bunch of chronic complainers that one best kept away from one's practice.

In the 1970s and 1980s, a number of psychologists and psychiatrists disregarded Jacobson's advice and developed different behavioral and psychotherapeutic approaches to deal specifically with insomnia. These strategies were gradually refined and improved until, in a conference on insomnia at Stanford in December 1988, the consensus was that at least three of every four chronic insomniacs could be helped quite markedly with psychological and behavioral treatment techniques.

Unfortunately, much of the good new work that has been done on insomnia is either not published or published in specialty journals not available to the general mental health professional. I felt that there was a need to bring all the different approaches on insomnia together, and I hope that this book will fill that need. I invited most of the leading insomnia specialists in the United States to describe their approaches to insomnia, and I asked them to do this in steps that can be followed by any trained professional. Most agreed to help with this project.

Although many authors in this book are identified with specific techniques, in clinical practice, most of us are quite eclectic, tailoring parts of different techniques to the needs of the individual patient. My main difficulty as the editor of this book was to keep each author from covering the entire field of possible treatments of insomnia, to keep the contributions distinct and focused on the specific area in which each author was an authority. Nevertheless, it is easily apparent in this book that the time of using only one narrow technique or one narrow school of thought has passed. One needs to be proficient in a wide variety of treatment approaches to insomnia and adapt the different techniques to the individual patient's needs.

Although the individual techniques may be widely different among those who treat insomnia, the patients we all see are about the same. This book, therefore, emphasizes the case study method, the time-honored practice to teach and to learn by discussing individual patients. However, we go one step further. Each author was asked not only to present a successful case, but also an unsuccessful one. Successful cases show a given method at its best and they illustrate how the technique should work ideally. However, we often learn more from our unsuccessful cases if we study them carefully. They teach us the limits of our techniques, the theoretical flaws in our understanding, and the complexities of our patients.

Studying insomnia treatment by the case method does not mean that each new patient has to be approached in a totally new idiosyncratic way. In Chapter One, Spielman and Glovinsky struggle with the task of finding common threads and building a conceptual framework for insomnia. Finding common themes in insomnia has direct practical effects. The unwieldy array of clinical presentations can be better understood, and both diagnostic and treatment efforts are thereby enhanced. Spielman and Glovinsky's contribution brings structure and order into our thinking about insomnia, and their discussion of predisposing, precipitating, and perpetuating factors has benefited the field tremendously.

This book tries to accurately reflect the current state of knowledge and skill. It does not present a united, common point where controversies remain unresolved. One controversy is the question of the use of hypnotic medication. If an insomniac came to, say, Bootzin, he would not receive any hypnotics. If he came to me, he would likely receive a few pills for occasional, special nights, and if he came to Stepanski, he might get a hypnotic every night for a month. Listen to what each author says and make up your own mind. Similarly, some of us are strictly behavioral, others search for underlying psychological causes. Some send most insomniacs for a sleep study before they treat, others do this rarely or never. Only time will tell what is best for each type of insomniac.

This book is written for mental health practioners, including family practitioners, psychiatrists, psychologists, social workers, nurses, and others. Prerequisites for using these techniques and approaches are clinical skills in interviewing, in treating mental and physical problems in general, and some training in the rudiments of supportive psychotherapy.

Note that this book is written for the professional. It is not a self-help book. It will be very difficult to apply what you learn in this book to your own case if you, yourself, have insomnia.

Together with the other authors, I sincerely hope that this book goes beyond a mere "how-to-do-it" cookbook, and that it helps you to understand the foundations of insomnia treatment. Summarizing the different techniques and approaches, it also imparts hope. Insomnia is no longer a chronic condition without treatment. It takes time and skill and patience, but most insomniacs today are treatable.

Peter J. Hauri, Ph.D.

Rochester, Minnesota

Contents

Chapter One
Introduction 1
Arthur J. Spielman and Paul B. Glovinsky

Part One
Specific Behavioral Techniques

Chapter Two
Stimulus Control Instructions 19
Richard R. Bootzin, Dana Epstein, and James M. Wood

Chapter Three
Stimulus Control in a Group Setting 29
Patricia Lacks

Chapter Four
Sleep Restriction Therapy 49
Paul B. Glovinsky and Arthur J. Spielman

Chapter Five
Sleep Hygiene, Relaxation Therapy, and Cognitive
Interventions 65
Peter J. Hauri

Part Two
Psychotherapeutic Techniques and Pharmacotherapy

Chapter Six
Insomnia: Psychotherapy or Not? 87
Vincent P. Zarcone, Jr.

Chapter Seven
Short-Term Psychotherapy for Chronic Insomnia 103
Andrew J. Borson

Chapter Eight
Pharmacotherapy of Insomnia 115
Edward J. Stepanski, Frank J. Zorick, and Thomas Roth

Part Three
Comprehensive and Integrated Approaches

Chapter Nine
Selecting a Treatment Strategy 133
Michael M. Stevenson and Marsha K. Weinstein

Chapter Ten
Breaking the Vicious Circle of Insomnia: A Treatment Model 155
Neil Steinberg

Chapter Eleven
Sleep Behavior Management 175
Sidney D. Nau, John H. Koewler, and James K. Walsh

Part Four
Disorders of the Sleep–Wake Schedule

Chapter Twelve
Assessment and Treatment of Delayed Sleep Phase Syndrome ... 193
Russell Rosenberg

Chapter Thirteen
Early Morning Awakening Insomnia: Bright-Light Treatment 207
Richard P. Allen

Part Five
Specific Populations

Chapter Fourteen
Insomnia in the Chronically Ill 223
Merrill M. Mitler, Steven Poceta, Stuart J. Menn,
and Milton K. Erman

Chapter Fifteen
Insomnia in the Older Adult 237
Judith Flaxman

Index 249

CHAPTER 1

Introduction
The Varied Nature of Insomnia

ARTHUR J. SPIELMAN AND PAUL B. GLOVINSKY

INTRODUCTION

Chronic insomnia has a profound impact on the quality of life. The transient variety is common enough to assure that most people will nod knowingly at the list of deficits this problem produces. Reduced zest, alertness, physical stamina, concentration, good-naturedness, enjoyment, and productivity are all reported. Experienced in a cascade, these impairments produce a general sense of vulnerability and disorder.

Substantial progress has been made in the diagnosis and treatment of insomnia (Association of Sleep Disorders Centers, 1979). Investigators and sleep disorders clinicians have shown that a careful diagnostic work-up, which may include all-night polysomnographic sleep recording, will often uncover features that direct specific treatment approaches (Edinger, Hoelscher, Webb, Marsh, Radtke, & Erwin, 1989). The informed clinician is no longer limited either to a symptomatic approach, employing hypnotics and analgesics, or to insight-oriented therapies intended for psychological disorders. Treatment modalities now include a range of behavioral approaches as well.

An understanding of insomnia is elusive because the condition arises from an interaction of factors. One patient's sleep maintenance insomnia

---

Arthur J. Spielman and Paul B. Glovinsky • Department of Psychology, The City College of the City University of New York, New York, New York 10031, and Insomnia Treatment Center, New York, New York 10017.

appears clearly reactive to job tensions. These ease on Friday and Saturday nights, leading to weekend oversleeping and a circadian disruption. As a result of the phase delay (later to bed and later to rise) over the weekend, sleep onset difficulties are added to the picture early in the week. A second patient readily traces the onset of his or her insomnia to a divorce ten years earlier, and indeed continues to dwell on this trauma during the day. However, while lying awake in bed at night, the content of his or her ruminations is exclusively concerned with the fear of sleeplessness and the daytime deficits that will follow. In these cases, both the obvious precipitants of insomnia, and the more subtle maintaining factors, appear relevant and may require specific attention. Ranking the importance of these multiple contributions remains problematic; in practice, treatment can become a series of trial-and-error explorations.

The treatments for such a multifaceted and mutable problem are themselves varied. Some treatments work on brain receptors, some on tense muscles. Some attempt to change how insomniacs perceive themselves and their sleep, while others attempt to change how they perceive their bedrooms. Some keep the insomniac in bed despite wakefulness, and some boot the patient out.

What is surprising, given this tangled state of affairs, is that our treatments work as well as they do. In this chapter, we will attempt to explore beneath the descriptive level with the purpose of identifying conceptual themes that clarify the workings of insomnia. Even a reduction of this sort will yield a list too long to treat appropriately here. We will, therefore, opt to focus on the following major themes: permitting sleep to occur; associative control of sleep; sleep drive, activation, and responsivity; the timing of sleep; the perception of sleep; and predisposing, precipitating, and perpetuating factors in insomnia.

PERMITTING SLEEP TO OCCUR

Sleep cannot be produced by force of will. All we can do is position ourselves to let it overtake us, like a surfer waiting for a wave. Fortunately, the waves come regularly: a defining characteristic of normal sleep is its recurrence at relatively equal intervals. The difficulty our patients have in falling asleep suggests the presence of barriers that interfere with the timely progression into sleep.

A number of barriers have been identified. Both cognitive activation and muscle tension can serve as obstacles to sleep. Racing thoughts, excitement over some prospect, or fear of yet another sleepless night can also suffice to keep us from sleeping. In fact, sleep is rather easily denied.

INTRODUCTION

Commonly seen are patients who report with chagrin how they can reach the verge of sleep, through relaxation, distraction, or sheer exhaustion, only to be pulled back into fretful wakefulness by fleeting thoughts or sounds outside their windows.

The fact that arousal should take precedence over sleep makes sense from an evolutionary perspective. No matter how important sleep may be, it was adaptively deferred when the mountain lion entered the cave. The problem, as Hauri (1989) has stressed, is that the time course of arousal is rapid, while the time course of dearousal is slow. It takes less than a second to be frightened by that ghastly apparition standing not ten feet from the bed, but when we then realize that it is really an overcoat on a rack, the damage is already done. The heart is pounding, the limbs are tensed, and it will be many minutes before physiology returns to a state that would permit sleep. Insomniacs are particularly adept at creating "apparitions," using, not overcoats, but meetings scheduled for first thing in the morning or recently committed blunders, to the same effect.

Psychopathology is common in individuals with sleep disturbance (Kales, Caldwell, Preston, Healey, & Kales, 1976; Mellinger, Balter, & Uhlenhuth, 1985; Ford & Kamerow, 1989). Research has shown that about one-third of individuals presenting with insomnia at sleep disorders centers also have concurrent psychiatric disorders (Coleman, et al., 1982). Similarly, there is a high prevalence of insomnia among psychiatric patients (Sweetwood, Kripke, Grant, Yager, & Gerst, 1976). However, the connection between psychopathology and insomnia is far from invariant; many patients with severe psychiatric disorders sleep well, and a large proportion of patients with insomnia do not have psychiatric disorders.

A recent longitudinal study of insomnia and psychopathology has shown that when insomnia resolves, the probability of new major depression is reduced (Ford & Kamerow, 1989). Given these results and the advances in the diagnosis and therapy of insomnia, clinicians should be encouraged to aggressively attend to the insomnia disorders. Although insomnia may often be part of a psychological disorder, the attitude that insomnia need not be directly addressed because treatment of the emotional problem is necessary and sufficient for a satisfactory outcome is outdated. We suggest that a view more in line with current understanding would appreciate the effectiveness of specific treatments for insomnia and the psychological prophylaxis such treatment affords.

The mechanisms by which psychiatric problems lead to sleep disturbances are far from clear, although manifest cognitive and physiological arousal may play a role (Freedman & Sattler, 1982; Lichstein & Rosenthal, 1980; Monroe, 1967; Nicassio, Mendlowitz, Fussell, & Petras, 1985). A number of studies have been conducted that serve as experimental analogues of the sleep disturbance associated with psychopathology. The sleep disturbance associated with the first night spent in a sleep lab may be due to uncertainty, increased scanning of the environment, and a general increase in cognitive activity (Agnew, Webb, & Williams, 1966). These same psychological factors may be present at home in the case of the insomniac with an anxiety disorder. Similarly, a study that manipulated cognitive intrusions showed that a group expected to give a three-minute speech on a specific topic after awakening from a nap had a harder time falling asleep than a control group (Gross & Borkovec, 1982). Likewise, the administration of stimulant drugs, such as nicotine and caffeine, may mimic the physiological arousal of an anxiety state and increase sleep latency and reduce sleep duration (Karacan, Thornby, Anch, Booth, Williams, & Salis, 1976; Soldatos, Kales, Scharf, Bixler, & Kales, 1980).

A number of behavioral treatments focus on dampening cognitive and physiological activation in order to permit sleep to occur. Relaxation training, biofeedback, and hypnotic imagery all fall into this category. While such exercises may be practiced for extended periods, their efficacy may reside in their ability to maintain a quiescent state for the ten minutes or so needed for sleep to overtake us. In other words, it may not be necessary to demolish barriers to sleep—just to lower them for a short while when sleep is about to overtake us.

ASSOCIATIVE CONTROL OF SLEEP

In contrast to the preceding viewpoint that stresses the importance of conditions within the organism in permitting sleep behavior, a learning perspective suggests that sleep behavior can be regulated by particular stimulus conditions. Sterman and colleagues, for example, demonstrated classical conditioning of sleep in cats (Sterman, Clemente, & Wyrwicka, 1963). They first showed that electrical stimulation of the preoptic basal forebrain rapidly produced sleep. They then used this stimulation as an unconditioned stimulus (UCS), pairing it with a tone, the conditioned stimulus (CS), in a classical conditioning paradigm. By the 38th trial, the tone itself produced slowing in the electroencephalogram (EEG). Further trials produced the rapid onset of behavioral sleep following the tone. Sleep became a conditioned response (CR). Further trials employing a tone of a different frequency and electrical stimulation of an arousing brain site demonstrated the learning principles of generalization and discrimination conditioning.

Bootzin discussed the associative process in humans, describing how environmental stimuli gain control of sleep behavior (Bootzin & Nicassio,

1978). The basis of this model is the well-known control of behavior that accrues to stimulus conditions in the course of discrimination conditioning. In good sleepers, cues such as the proper pillow or pre-sleep rituals such as tooth-brushing are repeatedly associated with rapid sleep onset. Cues such as talking excitedly on the telephone, watching stimulating television programs, and planning the next day's challenges do not occur in the bedroom, so that the ensuing arousal is not associated with the sleeping environment or pre-sleep rituals. In this way, these two different sets of cues actually gain control over the appearance of either sleep behavior or arousing behavior. With the onset of insomnia, however, bedroom cues may be repeatedly paired with agitation rather than sleep. The repeated pairing of bedroom cues and tossing and turning produces a maladaptive association, and the bedroom cues lead to agitation; sleeplessness results. Engaging in behaviors that are incompatible with sleep in bed is another route by which the bedroom cues may acquire arousing properties. Eating, talking on the telephone, doing homework, and watching the news in bed may establish a connection between the arousal that results from these behaviors and the cues of the bed and bedroom. Stimulus control instructions (Bootzin & Nicassio, 1978), discussed in Chapters Two and Three aim to reestablish bedroom cues as discriminative cues for rapid sleep onset.

Conditioning also appears to play an important role with respect to the pharmacological promotion of sleep. Recent research in animals indicates that associative mechanisms modulate tolerance (Siegel, 1975). If these findings are replicated in humans, it would suggest that contextual cues relating to sleeping pill usage—the room in which they are swallowed, the glass of water, the shape of the pill—are important determinants of tolerance to the drug.

It has consistently been demonstrated in animal studies that tolerance can be augmented or attenuated through the manipulation of the contextual cues previously associated with drug delivery (King, Bouton, & Musty, 1987; Siegel, 1975). Although procedures differed, in general, different groups received identical drug exposure and the group tested in the environment in which the drug was previously administered demonstrated greater tolerance. According to one theory, based on classical conditioning, repeated association of the environmental cues surrounding drug ingestion with the drug effects, a response antagonistic to the drug effect is learned (Siegel, 1975). Tolerance is understood to be the combination of the drug effect and the opposing learned response. One way to test whether the learned response is opposite to the drug effect is to present all of the cues previously associated with the drug delivery but omit the drug.

In an animal study pairing environmental cues with the sedating benzodiazepine midazolam (King *et al.*, 1987) for example, once tolerance had developed, a trial in which the environmental cues were followed by saline resulted in hyperactivity. Thus, what appeared to be learned was hyperactivity, a response antagonistic to the direct drug effect. The classical conditioning theory proposes that tolerance is the net effect of combining the direct response to the drug with the antagonistic conditioned response.

In addition to elucidating the importance of associative processes in the modulation of sleep, a conditioning perspective suggests ways in which to retard the development of drug tolerance by delivering placebo to reduce conditioned tolerance (Spielman, Caruso, & Glovinsky, 1987a). Such strategies may eventually improve the drug treatment of insomnia.

SLEEP DRIVE, ACTIVATION, AND RESPONSIVITY

Whether or not an individual will sleep can be conceptualized as dependent on several independent factors. The physiological drive to sleep may be relatively high or low. An opposing tendency to maintain alertness may arise from cortical excitation or other physiological sources. These two factors are clearly subject to fluctuations, although they tend to operate within a range of values for an individual. In addition to this shifting balance of sleep and activation, the individual also displays a characteristic level of responsiveness. Psychological characteristics contribute to the probability of a response or the magnitude of the response to a given stimulus. The lowered auditory arousal threshold to hearing one's own name provides an example of this psychological dimension.

A simple model, presented for its heuristic value, can be constructed to illustrate the interaction of three factors—sleep, activation, and responsiveness—in determining the sleep disturbance threshold (see Figure 1). This threshold is defined as the intensity of noise, worry, or any other stimulus, sufficient to inhibit sleep or cause more than momentary arousal.

The resolution of the sleep drive and the opposing activation level is one of the major determinants of the sleep disturbance threshold. A resolution in line with a larger sleep drive, Figure 1(4) compared to 1(2), for example, results in a higher sleep disturbance threshold and, hence, more robust sleep; sleep latency shortens, sleep duration lengthens, there are fewer sleep stage changes, there is a higher auditory arousal threshold, and nocturnal awakenings are shorter.

Sleep loss increases sleep drive, thus raising the sleep disturbance threshold. The initial phase of sleep restriction therapy, with its rapidly

INTRODUCTION

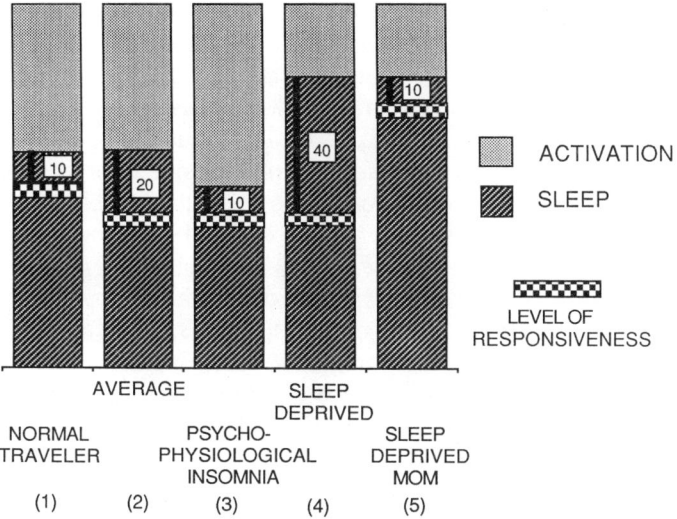

Figure 1. The sleep disturbance threshold, defined as the difference between the interaction of sleep and activation levels and the level of responsiveness, is depicted in five situations. This threshold is the intensity of any stimulus sufficient to inhibit sleep or cause a more than momentary arousal. For these situations we have used the auditory arousal threshold during sleep as the measure corresponding to the sleep disturbance threshold. (1) Normal sleep and activation levels with an increased responsiveness—this individual is trying to get up early to make a crucial travel connection, 10 decibels required; (2) normal sleep and activation levels with an average set point of responsiveness—20 decibels required to produce an awakening; (3) psychophysiological insomnia—a somewhat reduced sleep drive and increased activation level yield a lower sleep disturbance threshold of 10 decibels; (4) sleep deprivation—increased sleep drive and decreased activation yield an increased sleep disturbance threshold of 40 decibels: (5) sleep-deprived new mother—increased sleep drive and decreased activation combined with an increased responsiveness yield a lower sleep disturbance threshold of 10 decibels.

accumulating sleep debt, will tend to ameliorate sleep disturbance regardless of other factors that may be present (Spielman, Saskin, & Thorpy, 1987b). If insomnia stems directly from a low sleep drive, therapy will consist of titrating enough sleep loss into the system to promote sleep at night without introducing an unacceptable level of sleepiness during the day. If, as is probably more often the case, numerous factors in addition to a relatively low drive are contributing to the problem, patients should still improve under sleep restriction, and in fact be open to a host of ancillary benefits. The therapy's promotion of rapid sleep onset will strengthen associative cues at bedtime. It will reduce night-to-night variability in total sleep time, giving patients less cause for concern over what the night will bring. It establishes rigorous scheduling of sleep, thereby reinforcing circadian organization. As these benefits accrue, time in bed is increased to a level where sleep loss ceases to play an active role.

Similarly, hypnotic drug therapies for insomnia may directly augment sleep propensity for patients whose low drive for sleep is a sufficient cause of their insomnia. In these individuals, administration of a hypnotic would constitute more than merely symptomatic relief—it would represent a direct remedy for pathophysiology.

Ontogenetic changes resulting in a reduced depth of sleep may result in some elderly patients who have essentially lost an adequate drive for sleep. Again, the goal of therapy might be to reestablish a better equilibrium between activation and sleep drive by heightening sleep propensity, and hypnotics or mild sleep deprivation may be appropriate interventions.

The role of physiological activation in inhibiting sleep [see Figure 1(3)] has been demonstrated in insomniacs and in uncomplaining subjects undergoing experimental manipulations. Autonomic measures of activation, such as body temperature, heart rate, and galvanic skin response, have been reported elevated in "poor sleepers" (Monroe, 1967); some of these findings were replicated in insomniacs (Freedman & Sattler, 1982). Stimulants are also clearly capable of disturbing sleep, whether ingested through beverages, cigarettes, or medications.

Recent work investigating the sleepiness/alertness continuum (Seidel, Ball, Cohen, Patterson, Yost, & Dement, 1984) has suggested that insomniacs have increased daytime activation. A subgroup of insomniacs had no sleep propensity on a standard objective measure of daytime sleepiness. Another study (Stepanski, Zorick, Roehrs, Young, & Roth, 1988) found a counterintuitive relationship between nocturnal sleep and daytime sleepiness in insomniacs: those with the least amount of sleep at night were also the most highly activated during the day.

Although the model posits independent factors of sleep drive and activation level, the currently available measures of sleep, such as sleep latency, sleep duration, and arousal threshold, and waking function, such as mood, performance, and alertness, represent the interaction of these two factors. Therefore, with current methods, it is difficult to separate the effects of sleep loss or hypnotic drugs on the sleep drive from their impact on activation level.

Another factor, the level of responsiveness, enters into the equation alongside sleep drive and activation level in determining the sleep disturbance threshold. The model assumes that responsiveness may be changed independently of the other two factors. Motivation, for example, may affect responsiveness and result in a lowered sleep disturbance threshold.

The new mother's exquisite responsiveness to her infant's nocturnal distress, despite chronic sleep loss, provides one common example of psychological meaningfulness modulating the sleep disturbance threshold [Figure 1(5)]. Although the soldier on the battlefield may want to go to sleep, fear and vigilance increase the sleep disturbance threshold and sleep onset will be inhibited. The traveler's desire to awaken extremely early so as not to miss a crucial connection is successful owing to this change in responsivity affecting the threshold [Figure 1(1)].

In sleep maintenance insomnia, a bundle of conflicts may substitute for the baby. The insomniac may be primed to respond to these conflicts, continually scanning the internal environment just as the mother continues her vigilance over events in the crib even while asleep. In these cases, the individual has reset his or her responsivity based on the relative risks and rewards of going to sleep or sleeping through a pressing event.

The setting of a subjective response criterion in this manner is analogous to other decisions generally analyzed through signal detection theory. For example, a radar operator will decide whether or not a blip merits an all-hands alert based on what he perceives to be the risk of missing an enemy plane versus the reproach that would accompany a false alarm. The insomniac may have relatively more numerous "blips" to begin with, in the form of worries, hurts, and anxieties, and may attach greater risk to leaving those "blips" unattended.

In this model of insomnia, sleep disturbance threshold is therefore determined by subjectively assigned meanings, as well as the compromise between opposing physiological tendencies.

THE TIMING OF SLEEP

"When will I fall asleep?" and "How early will I wake-up?" are common concerns of most insomniacs. Potentially relevant to the insomniac with trouble falling asleep are studies of uncomplaining sleepers on ultrashort sleep–wake cycles and during nonentrained conditions when there is a lack of synchronization between the sleep–wake and body temperature rhythms (Lavie, 1986; Strogatz, Kronauer, & Czeisler, 1987).

It has been found that it is very difficult to fall asleep two to four hours before the beginning of the nocturnal propensity for sleep; this window of time has been called a "forbidden zone" or a "wake–maintenance zone." Remarkably, this zone was not eliminated by sleep deprivation (Lavie, 1986). It has been suggested that the individual with sleep onset difficulties may have a small phase delay so that the evening "wake-maintenance zone" is now occurring at the time that the individual is trying to fall asleep. This mechanism has also been invoked to explain the difficulties in falling asleep on Sunday night experienced by people who have allowed their circadian phases to drift later by going to sleep and arising later over the weekend.

Sleep-onset insomniacs studied during activities of general living and in experimental paradigms designed to minimize the exogenous influence on the phase of circadian rhythms have shown this hypothesized phase delay (Lack, Balfour, & Kalucy, 1985; MacFarlane, Cleghorn, Brown, Kaplan, Brown, & Mittorn, 1984; Morris, Lack, & Dawson, 1990). The four-hour delay discovered in the insomniacs' temperature rhythms (Morris, Lack, & Dawson, 1990) means that their habitual bedtimes fall within the wake-maintenance zone and may be the pathophysiological underpinnings of the sleep difficulty.

Circadian rhythm factors also contribute to premature sleep offset. Studies during desynchronized free-running conditions have shown that when subjects chose to go to sleep at a time when their body temperature rhythms were at or near their lowest values, sleep was short (Czeisler, Weitzman, Moore-Ede, Zimmerman, & Knauer, 1980). In other words, because subjects tend to wake up as the temperature rhythms are rising, going to sleep as the temperature rhythms are starting to rise (at the temperature minima) leads to short sleep. Individuals in normal 24-hour conditions may also have sleep durations governed by circadian rhythm factors. On nights when individuals go to sleep hours later than usual because of shiftwork or westward jet travel, they may be unable to maintain an adequate sleep duration, because of the arousing effects of the underlying circadian oscillator.

Recent work demonstrates that exposure to bright light, without changing the timing of the sleep–wake schedule, shifts the phase of the body temperature rhythm. This line of work, discussed in Chapters Twelve and Thirteen, suggests potential treatment strategies to help deal with misaligned rhythms (Czeisler *et al.*, 1986).

THE PERCEPTION OF SLEEP

It is common knowledge that insomniacs' subjective reports of sleep generally do not correspond to objective measures of sleep. However, insomniacs' estimates do faithfully reflect the severity of the sleep problems (Carskadon, Dement, Mitler, Guilleminault, Zarcone, & Spiegel, 1976). Those insomniacs complaining of long sleep latencies or short sleep are suffering from more severe sleep disturbances than insomniacs with reports of less disturbed sleep; however, there is a group of patients whose subjective assessment of sleep is so extreme that it rivets one's attention. These individuals report no sleep at all for many days, weeks, or months on end. We have polysomnographically studied a number of such patients, and, in all cases, there was substantial polygraphically recorded sleep at night associated with the morning subjective report of "no sleep." In these cases, the utility of the objective measures traditionally employed is suspect. The measures may not be sensitive to sleep characterized by ruminative self-monitoring. Of course, we must acknowledge that only a fraction of the data derived from the sleep recording is considered. Although some as yet undescribed combination of these parameters or EEG waveform analysis may be the culprit, the lack of a clue, given the extent of the complaint, remains a puzzle to sleep clinicians.

PREDISPOSING, PRECIPITATING, AND PERPETUATING FACTORS

We close this chapter by presenting a scheme we use to categorize and prioritize the factors contributing to insomnia and help in the development of a treatment plan. Insomnia is seen as the end result of predisposing, precipitating, and perpetuating factors (Spielman, 1986). Precipitating factors are flushed out by the question "Why now?" All clinicians are trained to elicit them, and they often provide sufficient information to formulate an initial treatment: Kick the newly acquired dog out of the bed. Don't linger over cappuccino just because a place opened down the block. See if the problem persists after the priority score of your grant is announced.

The other two factors are more easily overlooked. Predisposing factors are conditions that set the stage or determine the threshold for insomnia. A weak sleep-generating system may be a predisposing factor. A history of recurrent depression, the predilection to stay up late and sleep late ("owlishness"), or a susceptibility to anxiety states may also predispose to insomnia.

Perpetuating factors are generally not present during the inception of insomnia but make their appearance as a consequence of coping with the problem. They include both mental states and behavioral practices. Here is our roundup of the usual suspects:

1. Excessive time in bed
2. Irregular timing of retiring and arising
3. Unpredictability of sleep
4. Anxiety over daytime deficits

5. Expectation of a bad night
6. Fragmentation of sleep
7. Maladaptive conditioning
8. Caffeine consumption
9. Hypnotic and alcohol ingestion

We can trace the changing composition of factors leading to insomnia over time (see Figure 2). Assume that a young man had owlish tendencies to which he had adapted reasonably well (premorbid). A promotion brings new job responsibilities, closer scrutiny, and the development of an anxiety state. The combination exceeds the threshold for insomnia (acute insomnia). He then begins to catch up on sleep over the weekends, when the pressure is off, and to worry about decreased job performance caused by sleep loss (early insomnia). By the time he comes to clinical attention, he may have the job pretty much under control, but the insomnia persists (chronic insomnia).

Note that at this point, addressing our patient's propensity for delayed sleep may be insufficient to produce improvement; however, once sleep hygiene measures and more specific treatments have been introduced, long-term management would benefit from recommendations aimed at preventing a sleep phase delay.

The oft heard lament "nothing is bothering me except that I worry about my insomnia" may become the central feature maintaining a sleep disturbance. Insomnia produced by stress and major life events makes

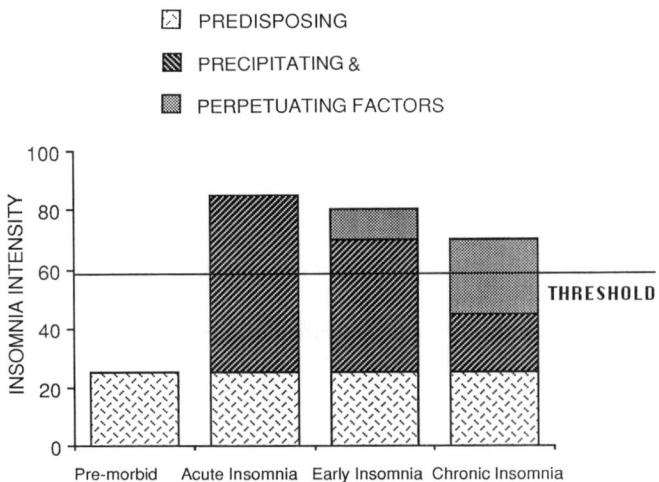

Figure 2. Factors contributing to the development of insomnia. Effective treatment and long-term management of insomnia require one to address these separate influences.

intuitive sense; the dimensions of the problem or excitement produce sufficient cognitive arousal to interfere with sleep. As events fade, or stress is adapted to, the insomnia wanes; however, in some individuals the self-attribution "I am an insomniac," the expectation of a bad night, the anticipation of the discomfort of a sleepless night, or the dread of daytime deficits is in and of itself arousing. The subsequent sleep disturbance completes the vicious cycle: anxious worry → sleep disturbance → anxious worry → . . . Effective treatment of any type will help interrupt this cycle; however, it is only when the patient forestalls the next bout of insomnia with the techniques he or she has learned, gaining confidence and a sense of mastery, that this insidious cycle is broken.

CONCLUSION

It is our belief that formulations based on a conceptual approach yield direct practical benefits; the unwieldy array of clinical presentations of insomnia can be grasped, and both diagnostic and treatment efforts enhanced. Insomnia perplexes both clinicians and patients because its very nature is elusive; often it is symptomatic of an underlying physical, psychological, or circadian rhythm disorder, sometimes it derives from the individual's inherent physiological makeup, and it may be maintained by practices specifically initiated to cope with the problem. Therefore, careful assessment, reasoned formulation, appropriate treatment, and close monitoring of the patient for compliance are all necessary to deal effectively with the challenge of insomnia.

Arthur J. Spielman is Professor of Psychology, Head of the Experimental Cognition Doctoral Program, and Director of the Sleep Disorders Center at the City College of the City University of New York. He is a clinical psychologist and an accredited clinical polysomnographer with experience in the research, evaluation, and treatment of sleep disorders, specializing in the behavioral treatment of insomnia. Dr. Spielman was previously Co-Director of the Sleep–Wake Disorders Center at Montefiore Medical Center and is currently Co-Director of the Insomnia Treatment Center in New York City.

Paul B. Glovinsky received his Ph.D. in Clinical Psychology from the City College of the City University of New York, where he is currently an Adjunct Assistant Professor in the Experimental Cognition Doctoral Program. Dr. Glovinsky has investigated mechanisms of daytime sleepiness, narcolepsy, and clinical and theoretical issues of insomnia. An accredited clinical polysomnographer, he was staff psychologist at the Montefiore Medical Center's Sleep–Wake Disorders Center for several years and is currently Co-Director of the Insomnia Treatment Center in New York City.

RECOMMENDED READINGS

Bootzin, R. R. & Nicassio, P. M. (1978). Behavioral treatments for insomnia. In: *Progress in behavior modification* (Vol. 6). New York: Academic Press, pp. 1–45.
A thorough review of the empirical work on insomnia up to 1978, this paper also includes a number of behavioral studies that are quite suggestive yet less well known.

Hauri, P. (1982). *The sleep disorders*. Kalamazoo, MI: Upjohn. A Scope Publication.
A primer that presents a well-proportioned frame of reference to all the sleep disorders.

Spielman, A. J., Caruso, L., & Glovinsky, P. B. (1987a). A behavioral perspective on insomnia treatment. In: M. Ermin (Ed.), *Psychiatric clinics of North America*. Philadelphia: W. B. Saunders, pp. 541–553.
Although some material in the present chapter appears in this earlier work, a description of the treatment methods complements the current work.

REFERENCES

Association of Sleep Disorders Centers. (1979). Diagnostic classification of sleep and arousal disorders (1st ed.). Prepared by the Sleep Disorders Classification Committee, H. P. Roffwarg, Chairman. *Sleep, 2*, 1–137.

Agnew, H. W., Webb, W. B., & Williams, R. L. (1966). The first-night effect: An EEG study of sleep. *Psychophysiology, 2*, 263–266.

Bootzin, R. R., & Nicassio, P. M. (1978). Behavioral treatments for insomnia. In *Progress in behavior modification* (Vol. 6). New York: Academic Press, pp. 1–45.

Carskadon, M. A., Dement, W. C., Mitler, M. M., Guilleminault, C., Zarcone, V. P., & Spiegel, R. (1976). Self-reports versus sleep laboratory fincings in 122 drug-free subjects with complaints of chronic insomnia. *American Journal of Psychiatry, 133*, 1382–1388.

Coleman, R., Roffwarg, H. P., Kennedy, S., et al. (1982). Sleep–wake disorders based on a polysomnoagraphic diagnosis: A national cooperative study. *Journal of the American Medical Association, 247*, 997–1003.

Czeisler, C. A., Weitzman, E. D., Moore-Ede, M. C., Zimmerman, J. C., & Knauer, R. (1980). Human sleep: Its duration and organization depend on its circadian phase. *Science, 210*, 1264–1267.

Czeisler, C. A., Allan, J. S., Strogatz, S. H., Ronda, J. M., Sanchez, R., Rios, C. D., Freitag, W. O., Richardson, G. S., & Kronauer, R. E. (1986). Bright light resets the human circadian pacemaker independent of the timing of the sleep-wake cycle. *Science 233*, 667–671.

Edinger, J. D., Hoelscher, T. J., Webb, M. D., Marsh, G. R., Radtke, R. A., & Erwin, C. W. (1989). Polysomnographic assessment of DIMS: Empirical evaluation of its diagnostic value. *Sleep, 12*(4), 315–322.

Ford, D. E., & Kamerow, D. B. (1989). Epidemiologic study of sleep disturbance and psychiatric disorders. *Journal of the American Medical Association, 262*(11), 1479–1484.

Freedman, R., & Sattler, H. (1982). Physiological and psychological factors in sleep-onset insomnia. *Journal of Abnormal Psychology, 91*, 380–389.

Gross, R. T., & Borkovec, T. D. (1982). Effects of a cognitive intrusion manipulation on the sleep-onset latency of good sleepers. *Behavior Therapy, 13*, 112–116.

Hauri, P. (1989). Primary insomnia. In *American Psychiatric Association treatments of psychiatric disorders: A task force report of the APA* (Vol. 3). Washington, DC: APA, pp. 2424–2433.

Kales, A., Caldwell, A. B., Preston, T. A., Healey, S., & Kales, J. D., (1976). Personality patterns in insomnia. *Archives of General Psychiatry, 33,* 1128–1134.

Karacan, I., Thornby, J. I., Anch, A. M., Booth, G. H., Williams, R. L., & Salis, P. J. (1976). Dose-related sleep disturbances induced by coffee and caffeine. *Clinical Pharmacology and Therapeutics, 20,* 682–689.

King, D. A., Bouton, M. E., & Musty, R. E. (1987). Associative control of tolerance to the sedative effects of a short-acting benzodiazepine. *Behavioral Neuroscience, 101,* 104–114.

Lack, L., Balfour, R., & Kalucy, R. (1985). The circadian rhythms of body temperature in poor sleepers. *Sleep Research, 14,* 298.

Lavie, P. (1986). Ultrashort sleep-waking schedule. III. "Gates" and "forbidden zones" for sleep. *Electroencephalographs and Clinical Neurophysiology, 63,* 414–425.

Lichstein, K. L., & Rosenthal, T. L. (1980). Insomniacs' perceptions of cognitive versus somatic determinants of sleep disturbance. *Journal of Abnormal Psychology, 89,* 105–107.

MacFarlane, J., Cleghorn, J. M., Brown, G. M., Kaplan, R., Brown, P., & Mittorn, J. (1984). *Sleep Research, 13,* 223.

Mellinger, G. D., Balter, M. B., & Uhlenhuth EH. (1985). Insomnia and its treatment: Prevalence and correlates. *Archives of General Psychiatry, 42,* 225–232.

Monroe, L. J. (1967). Psychological and physiological differences between good and poor sleepers. *Journal of Abnormal Psychology, 72,* 255–264.

Morris, M., Lack, L., & Dawson, D. (1990). Sleep-onset insomniacs have delayed temperature rhythms. *Sleep, 13*(1), 1–14.

Nicassio, P. M., Mendlowitz, D. R., Fussell, J. J., & Petras, L. (1985). The phenomenology of the pre-sleep state: The development of the Pre-Sleep Arousal Scale. *Behaviour Research and Therapy, 23,* 263–271.

Seidel, W. F., Ball, S., Cohen, S., Patterson, N., Yost, D., & Dement, W. C. (1984). Daytime alertness in relation to mood, performance, and nocturnal sleep in chronic insomniacs and noncomplaining sleepers. *Sleep, 7*(3), 230–238.

Siegel, S. (1975). Evidence from rats that morphine tolerance is a learned response. *Journal of Comparative and Physiological Psychology, 89,* 498–506.

Soldatos, C. R., Kales, J., Scharf, M. B., Bixler, E. O., & Kales, A. (1980). Cigarette smoking associated with sleep difficulty. *Science, 207,* 551–552.

Spielman, A. J. (1986). Assessment of insomnia. *Clinical Psychology Reviews, 6,* 11–25.

Spielman, A. J., Caruso, L., & Glovinsky, P. B. (1987a). A behavioral perspective on insomnia treatment. In M. Ermin (Ed.), *Psychiatric clinics of North America*. Philadelphia: W. B. Saunders, pp. 541–553.

Spielman, A. J., Saskin, P., & Thorpy, M. J. (1987b). Treatment of chronic insomnia by restriction of time in bed. *Sleep, 10*(1), 45–56.

Stepanski, E., Zorick, F., Roehrs, T., Young, D., & Roth, T. (1988). Daytime alertness, in patients with chronic insomnia compared with asymptomatic control subjects. *Sleep, 11*(1), 54–60.

Sterman, M. B., Clemente, C. D., & Wyrwicka, W. (1963). Forebrain inhibitory mechanisms: Conditioning of basal forebrain induced EEG synchronization and sleep. *Experimental Neurology, 7*(5), 404–417.

Strogatz, S. H., Kronauer, R. E., & Czeisler, C. A. (1987). Circadian pacemaker interferes with sleep onset at specific times each day: Role in insomnia. *American Physiological Society, 1987,* R172–R178.

Sweetwood, H. L., Kripke, D. F., Grant, I., Yager, J., & Gerst, M. S. (1976). Sleep disorder and psychobiological symptomatology in male psychiatric outpatients and male nonpatients. *Psychosomatics Medicine, 38,* 373–378.

Part One

Specific Behavioral Techniques

Part One introduces the special behavioral techniques used in the treatment of insomnia. In a very real sense, here you learn the "nuts and bolts" of what the behaviorist does when working with a case of sleeplessness. Each method is presented by the person who has either developed the technique or has done most research on it.

In developing these four chapters, my main problem was that nobody, not even the originators of these methods, uses them rigidly, in a vacuum. All emphasize the fact that behavioral methods must be adapted to the situation and to the patient. All talk to their patients and then decide what method might be most applicable.

Reviewing the individual chapters in this section, it is only fitting that we start with a chapter on stimulus control therapy. This approach, pioneered by Richard Bootzin, is probably the most powerful and most widely used treatment program for insomnia, and the one that has generated most research. Stimulus control instructions were derived directly from learning principles, they have a clear rationale, and extensive research has been carried out on them. This research shows convincingly that stimulus control techniques work at least as well as, if not better than, any other approaches to insomnia.

A very efficient and powerful extension of stimulus control therapy is its use in group treatment, as discussed in Chapter Three by Patricia Lacks. Combining stimulus control therapy with education about sleep, with sleep hygiene, and with sleep monitoring, Lacks has shown that four hours of treatment over a four-week period can cut in half the time a sleeper reports spending awake in bed. After four weeks, about one-third of her patients joined the ranks of good sleepers. Reading about Lacks's simple and straightforward approach, one wonders why group treatment of insomnia hasn't gained a larger following over the last few years.

Sleep restriction therapy is the topic of Chapter Four. This treatment of insomnia makes use of sleep deprivation to increase the drive to sleep. By doing so, it reduces sleep latency, consolidates sleep, and reduces night-by-night variability. Glovinsky and Spielman discuss not only the mechanics of this approach, but also the nuances of conducting behavioral treatments in general. They look at indications and contraindications of doing this kind of work, and they propose possible mechanisms of action.

Chapter Five first reviews sleep hygiene rules and how to individually apply them. These rules include curtailing the time one spends in bed, not trying desperately to fall asleep, eliminating the bedroom clock, exercising in the late afternoon, avoiding caffeine, alcohol, and nicotine, and so forth. Relaxation therapy is then explored: It appears that relaxation training helps many insomniacs and that the method by which one relaxes is less important than that relaxation be done very thoroughly. Finally, the therapist is invited to use the insomniac as a "coscientist," actively engaging the patient in the solution of his/her sleep problem rather than reinforcing a passive role.

CHAPTER TWO

Stimulus Control Instructions

RICHARD R. BOOTZIN, DANA EPSTEIN, AND JAMES M. WOOD

INTRODUCTION

The goals of stimulus control instructions are to help the insomniac learn to fall asleep quickly and to maintain sleep. These goals are reached by strengthening the bed as a cue for sleep, weakening it as a cue for activities that might interfere with sleep, and helping the insomniac acquire a consistent sleep rhythm. Although there are many causes of insomnia, poor sleep habits are often an important contributor.

Insomniacs often engage in activities at bedtime that are incompatible with falling asleep. They may, for example, use their bedrooms for reading, talking on the telephone, watching television, snacking, listening to music, or worrying. Many insomniacs seem to organize their entire existence around their bedroom, with television, telephone, books, and food within easy reach. For others, bedtime is the first available quiet time during the day to rehash the day's events and to worry and plan for the next day. Under these conditions, bed and bedtime become cues for arousal rather than for sleep.

Another cause of arousal for the insomniac is that the bedroom can become a cue for the anxiety and frustration associated with trying to fall asleep. Often insomniacs can sleep any place other than their own beds. They might fall asleep in easy chairs or on couches. They often have less difficulty sleeping when away from home, while normal sleepers often

---

Richard R. Bootzin, Dana Epstein, and James M. Wood • Department of Psychology, University of Arizona, Tucson, Arizona 85721.

have difficulty sleeping in strange surroundings. For normal sleepers, there are strong cues for sleep associated with their beds, and it is only when these cues are not available that they have difficulty.

INTAKE METHOD

Patients seen at the Insomnia Clinic of the University of Arizona Sleep Disorders Center take the Minnesota Multiphasic Personality Inventory (MMPI), provide medical and psychiatric histories, complete two weeks of daily sleep diaries, have thorough insomnia intake interviews, and, if it appears that other sleep disorders (e.g., sleep apnea, periodic leg movements) may contribute to the problem, have one- or two-night polysomnographic (PSG) studies. A one-night study is usually sufficient to identify sleep apnea and periodic leg movements; however, a two-night study may be necessary for patients who complain of getting almost no sleep at all. For such patients, two nights gives a better picture of the nature and quality of their sleep than does one. Approximately 20 percent of our patients are scheduled for PSGs, out of which about one-fourth are scheduled for two nights.

Daily sleep diaries are a critical component of our assessment and treatment process. The diary we employ contains entries for naps, sleep latency, number and duration of awakenings, total sleep, quality of sleep, and feelings upon awakening. The patients fill out the diaries each morning and use a comments column to note events that might have affected the night's sleep, such as the use of sleep medication, illness, emotional distress, or other unusual events.

Diaries are a practical, efficient means of obtaining information about the frequency of sleep problems in the patient's own environment (Bootzin & Engle-Friedman, 1981). As a consequence of keeping daily diaries, patients often find that their sleep problems are not as severe or as frequent as they thought. Daily diaries also provide a means of assessing whether or not interventions are having any effects. Without diaries, patients may become discouraged at the occurrence of single sleepless nights. Keeping sleep diaries helps to keep the patients focused on whether or not the frequency of the problems is changing.

An important first step for many patients we see is to help them withdraw from hypnotics. We work closely with the patients' prescribing physicians. For some patients, the hypnotics are maintaining the insomnia. In our experience, some patients' sleep improves substantially once they are medication free. A number of patients are so fearful of withdrawing from hypnotics that it is tempting to provide behavioral treatment while the patients are maintained on constant doses of hypnotics. Once the sleep problems have improved, the patients could be withdrawn from the hypnotics. Although this strategy often works initially, a dramatic worsening of sleep problems is associated with withdrawal (Espie, Lindsay, & Brooks, 1988). Patients need to be supported during this period, and behavioral treatment may need to be reinstituted following withdrawal. Because of the high frequency of drug dependence associated with benzodiazepines that we see in our clinic, we recommend against even the occasional use of hypnotics. It is our philosophy that it is more effective in the long run for patients to develop their own personal resources for dealing with insomnia than to depend on medication.

The approach at our Insomnia Clinic is to do a thorough assessment and to treat the sleep problem as comprehensively as possible. Any of the interventions described in other chapters might be employed for particular patients. Additionally, all patients are given information about sleep, such as the changes that occur with age and the effects on sleep of physical illness, prescription and nonprescription medication, alcohol, caffeine, nicotine, stress, inactivity, naps, and sleep environment factors. Stimulus control instructions serve as the core around which we build other components.

Stimulus Control Instructions

The following rules constitute the stimulus control instructions given to the patient (Bootzin, 1972, 1977). They form the foundation for the development of new permanent sleeping habits and are to be followed even after the insomniac is falling asleep faster and sleeping better.

1. Lie down intending to go to sleep *only* when you are sleepy.
2. Do not use your bed for anything except sleep; that is, do not read, watch television, eat, or worry in bed. Sexual activity is the only exception to this rule. On such occasions, the instructions are to be followed afterward when you intend to go to sleep.
3. If you find yourself unable to fall asleep, get up and go into another room. Stay up as long as you wish and then return to the bedroom to sleep. Although we do not want you to watch the clock, we want you to get out of bed if you do not fall asleep immediately. Remember that the goal is to associate your bed with falling asleep *quickly*! If you are in bed more than about ten minutes without falling asleep and have not gotten up, you are not following this instruction.

4. If you still cannot fall asleep, repeat rule 3. Do this as often as is necessary throughout the night.

5. Set your alarm and get up at the same time every morning irrespective of how much sleep you got during the night. This will help your body acquire a consistent sleep rhythm.

6. Do not nap during the day.

The focus of the instructions is primarily on sleep onset. Nevertheless, they can be used and have been found to be effective with sleep maintenance problems (e.g., Morin & Azrin, 1987). With sleep maintenance patients, the instructions are to be followed after awakening in the middle of the night.

Although the stimulus control instructions appear simple and straightforward, we have found that compliance is better if they are discussed individually and a rationale is provided for each rule. The rationales we discuss include the following:

Rule 1. The goal of this rule is help the patients become more sensitive to internal cues of sleepiness so that they will be more likely to fall asleep quickly when they go to bed.

Rule 2. The goals here are to have activities that are associated with arousal occur elsewhere and to break up patterns that are associated with disturbed sleep. If bedtime is the only time patients have for thinking about the day's events and planning for tomorrow, they should spend some quiet time doing that in another room before they go to bed. Many people without sleep problems read or listen to music in bed without problems, however, that is not the case for insomniacs. Thus, this instruction is used to help those who have sleep problems establish new routines to facilitate sleep.

Rules 3 and 4. In order to associate the bed with sleep and disassociate it from the frustration and arousal of not being able to sleep, the patients are instructed to get out of bed after about ten minutes (20 minutes for those over 60). This is also a means of coping with insomnia. By getting out of bed and engaging in other activities, patients are exerting control over their problems. The problems become more manageable and, as a consequence, less distress is experienced.

Rule 5. Insomniacs often have irregular sleep rhythms because they try to make up for poor sleep by sleeping late or by napping the next day. Keeping consistent wake times helps develop consistent sleep rhythms so that the patients will be more likely to be able to sleep at night. Additionally, the set wake times means that the patients will be somewhat sleep-deprived after a night of insomnia. This will make it more likely that the patients will fall asleep quickly the following night, strengthening the cues of the bed and bedroom for sleep.

Rule 6. The goal here is to keep insomniacs from disrupting their sleep patterns by irregular napping. A nap that takes places seven days a week at the same time would be permissible. For those elderly insomniacs who feel they need to nap, we recommend either a daily nap of less than an hour's length, or the use of 20 to 30 minutes of relaxation as a nap substitute.

Most of the problems involved in the patients' following through with stimulus control instructions can be solved by direct discussion with the patients. A common problem is the disturbance of the spouses' sleep when the insomniacs get out of bed. Discussions of the problem with the spouses are often helpful in ensuring full cooperation. During the winter in cold climates, some patients may be reluctant to leave the warmth of their beds. Suggestions for keeping warm robes near the beds and keeping an additional room warm through the night, along with encouragement to try to follow the instructions, are usually effective in promoting compliance (Bootzin, Engle-Friedman, & Hazelwood, 1983).

SUCCESSFUL CASE HISTORY

A good illustration of our approach occurred with a 31-year-old married woman (R) who experienced increasing difficulty sleeping, following the birth of her first child nine months earlier. When the child was seven months old, R experienced a period of ten days in which she reported that she did not sleep at all. Her physician prescribed 30 mg of temazepam, which worked effectively. After two weeks, the dose was reduced to 15 mg.

At the time of her interview at the Insomnia Clinic two months later, R was still taking 15 mg of temazepam each night but not sleeping well. Nevertheless, she believed that she needed the medication in order to sleep at all. Every time she had tried to go without it, she slept poorly, and she was afraid that she would have another long period of not sleeping at all if she stopped taking sleep medication.

A computerized diagnostic interview indicated that R met DSM-III (American Psychiatric Association, 1980) criteria for major depression. Although R met the formal criteria, the intensity of her depression was not severe, and, as will be discussed below, she had many personal resources. She reported that the following symptoms were present almost every day for a two-week period: loss of appetite, trouble sleeping, tired all the time, a lot more trouble concentrating, thoughts come more slowly or seem mixed up, frequent thoughts of death. She did not report suicidal thoughts, but rather that she had been thinking more philosophically about mortality since the birth of her child. Her MMPI indicated many complaints about depression and anxiety.

R had many personal resources. She was intelligent, articulate, and had a strong problem-solving orientation. Although treatment for depression was recommended, she rejected it, stating that she was convinced these were problems she could work on without professional help. She described a number of positive steps she was taking to add more enjoyment to her life. She was similarly determined to solve her sleep problems.

The first step of the treatment was to help her withdraw from temazepam. It was emphasized that the nights of sleeplessness she experienced when trying to do without medication were withdrawal effects and that she was going to have to stop taking hypnotics for a few weeks before seeing what her sleep was really like. First, she reduced her dose by half for a few days, and then she stopped taking it entirely.

Once R stopped taking hypnotics, her sleep did get worse temporarily. Stimulus control instructions had been explained and were to be used to help cope with sleeplessness caused by withdrawal and to develop a better sleep pattern. The instruction to get out of bed if she was having difficulty sleeping was particularly stressed. R's attempts to bring more enjoyment to her life were also supported. Within two weeks of stopping hypnotics, R's sleep consisted of a mix of three to four nights of poor sleep and three to four nights of good sleep. Over the next couple of weeks, the number of nights of sound sleep increased, until R was having only one night a week of poor sleep. At this point R concluded that she was capable of coping with an occasional poor night's sleep and she ended the therapy. A three-month telephone follow-up indicated that she continued to sleep well, with occasional poor nights, and that she was no longer depressed. It is somewhat surprising that R's depression improved along with her sleep. Usually, treatment needs to be directed at both the sleep and the emotional problems. In R's case, however, we may have caught her near the end of a depressive episode.

The stimulus control instructions were important in helping R cope with the withdrawal from hypnotics. There are a number of possible explanations for R's improved sleep:

1. The stimulus control instructions may have helped establish a better sleep pattern.
2. Once withdrawn from hypnotics, she experienced sleep patterns typical of her sleep before her child was born.
3. As her depression became more manageable, she slept better.
4. Her shift in attitude from that of being a victim of her sleep

problem to that of being able to cope with the problem reduced anxiety about sleep and produced improvement.

These explanations are not incompatible with one another. In a case study, it is not possible to disentangle alternative explanations, and all may have contributed to R's improvement.

CASE HISTORY OF A TREATMENT FAILURE

When seen by us, T was a 27-year-old, unemployed male who had recently moved from the East to live with his retired parents. He reported having severe sleep onset insomnia for the past eight years, beginning while he was away at college. Each night, one of his roommates would run up the stairs making loud noises. He began to anticipate the noises and found himself unable to sleep. T reported feeling intimidated by the roommate. The anticipatory anxiety about not sleeping developed into a common pattern in which the slightest change in environmental circumstances or the anticipation of stress the next day would lead to a sleepless night. T had difficulty keeping a job, which he attributed to his sleep problem and the resultant daytime sleepiness. T's daytime complaints included feelings of weakness and fatigue, blurred vision, depression, and panic attacks.

T's current problem centered around the morning garbage collection twice a week at his home. He reported not being able to fall asleep at all on the nights before the early-morning garbage collection because he anticipated being awakened by the noise. He reported hating to be disturbed once he finally fell asleep. It should be noted that he was never actually awakened by the garbage truck since it always came after he was up for the morning. Nevertheless, he feared it would come earlier and wake him up.

The computerized diagnostic interview indicated that T met the DSM-III criteria for both major depression and dysthymic disorder. T's MMPI indicated that he had many complaints about depression, anxiety, and somatization. Although T had many complaints of distress, this seemed to reflect a long-term personality style or personality disorder. His MMPI profile was similar to those seen in individuals who are judged to be immature, narcissistic, and demanding and for whom compliance with a treatment regimen is difficult.

T had been taking Dalmane and Xanax during the previous year. At the time he came to the Insomnia Clinic, he was under the care of a psychiatrist for his complaint of depression and had started taking Imipramine, 50 mg daily. He felt the Imipramine was keeping him awake and, at the suggestion of his psychiatrist, divided the daily dose between morning and night. T reported having had a PSG study while living in the East. He was asked to have the report sent to the Insomnia Clinic, but it never arrived.

Because T's sleep problem appeared related to long-standing psychological problems, continued treatment for depression and anxiety was recommended. We agreed to focus on T's sleep problem and his expectations about sleep and daytime functioning.

T was given daily sleep diaries to complete and told to restrict his sleep to the hours of 11 P.M. to 7 A.M. (the garbage collection occurred after 7 A.M.). Stimulus control instructions were discussed at the second session.

Throughout the treatment, sleep diaries were haphazardly completed. Often they were forgotten at home or in his car. Verbal reports from T made it clear that he was not following the stimulus control instructions despite his understanding of them. T would sleep on the couch the nights before garbage collection. He slept better on the couch because it was not near the side of the house from which the garbage was picked up.

Every treatment session dealt at considerable length with challenging unrealistic expectations and developing practical strategies for dealing with T's worries and anticipated stresses. Daytime activities were also discussed. It was emphasized that T needed to start being more active and productive in order to sleep better. He had instead been following the strategy of waiting for his sleep to improve before getting a job.

T's progress during treatment was highly variable. T would improve temporarily. At such times, he looked more alert and was in a good mood. There would be job prospects and his social life was improving. However, new difficulties and new bouts of severe insomnia recurred. He returned to obsessive worrying, sleeping on the couch, and episodes of anger directed primarily at his parents.

Throughout the time that T was seen in the Insomnia Clinic, he made numerous telephone calls to the therapist between sessions. He taped part of one session (at his suggestion) in order to help him identify self-defeating thoughts and to try to change his unrealistic expectations. Nevertheless, he frequently failed to show up for appointments or canceled them at the last minute. He continued to be both dependent and demanding. His parents paid his therapy bills, but usually after a considerable delay.

After about six months of treatment, T moved to the West Coast to take a job and live independently. He was given a referral to a sleep disorders center in his area. T continued to show the same cyclical pattern. He would improve briefly, but continued to have recurrent episodes of severe insomnia, often associated with environmental conditions such as traffic noise or excessive heat.

In T's case, his treatment needs were beyond the resources of the Insomnia Clinic. Stimulus control instructions and other behavioral treatments are primarily self-help treatments. They require the active cooperation of patients in carrying out assignments. T was unwilling or incapable of doing so. To be effective, treatment would have had to be directed at T's maladaptive personality style that caused problems with compliance.

DISCUSSION AND SUMMARY

The two cases presented here are representative of the range of patients who seek treatment for insomnia. Each individual has unique skills, deficits, and circumstances that call for individualization of treatment. It is essential, however, to use treatments that have been proven effective. Stimulus control therapy is such a treatment. It has been widely evaluated with insomniacs and appears to be the most effective nonpharmacological treatment of insomnia available today (e.g., Bootzin & Nicassio, 1978; Borkovec, 1982; Espie, Lindsay, Brooks, Hood, & Turvey, 1989). As illustrated in the case studies, stimulus control instructions can be a core component of individualized, multicomponent treatment.

Richard R. Bootzin received a Ph.D. in Clinical Psychology from Purdue University in 1968. He has been investigating behavioral approaches for insomnia since 1970. He was on the faculty of the Psychology Department of Northwestern University from 1968 through 1986. Currently, he is Professor of Psychology and Psychiatry at the University of Arizona, Director of the Graduate Program in Clinical Psychology, and Director of the Insomnia Clinic of the University of Arizona Sleep Disorders Center.

Dana Epstein received her M.A. in Nursing in 1987 from the University of Arizona and is currently a Ph.D. candidate in the College of Nursing at the University of Arizona. She has a special interest in sleep problems of the elderly and has worked with Dr. Bootzin in the Insomnia Clinic since 1988.

James M. Wood received a Ph.D. in Clinical Psychology from the University of Arizona in 1990. Currently, he is a postdoctoral fellow at the Palo Alto Veterans Administration Hospital in California. He worked with Dr. Bootzin in the Arizona Insomnia Clinic from 1988 through 1989.

RECOMMENDED READINGS

Bootzin, R. R., & Engle-Friedman, M. (1987). Sleep disturbances. In L. Carstensen & B. Edelstein (Eds.), *Handbook of clinical gerontology*. New York: Pergamon Press.

This chapter is particularly focused on sleep problems of the elderly. Detailed information is given on the assessment and behavioral treatment of insomnia in the elderly. Particular focus is given to stimulus control instructions, relaxation training, and sleep hygiene information.

Bootzin, R. R., & Nicassio, P. (1978). Behavioral treatments for insomnia. In M. Hersen, R. M. Eisler, and P. M. Miller (Eds.), *Progress in behavior modification* (Vol. 6). New York: Academic Press.

This is a thorough review of the rationales and evidence regarding a variety of behavioral techniques of insomnia. Although it is now over 12 years old, it is still a useful resource for identifying alternative behavioral techniques for the treatment of insomnia.

Lacks, P. (1987). *Behavioral treatment for persistent insomnia*. New York: Pergamon Press.

This is a very useful monograph on behavioral treatment of insomnia that gives a number of practical suggestions and includes a variety of assessment instruments. There is a detailed presentation of stimulus control instructions and how to implement them.

REFERENCES

American Psychiatric Association (1980). *Diagnostic and statistical manual of mental disorders* (3rd ed.). Washington, DC: American Psychiatric Association.

Bootzin, R. R. (1972). A stimulus control treatment for insomnia. *Proceedings of the American Psychological Association, 1972*, 395–396.

Bootzin, R. R. (1977). Effects of self-control procedures for insomnia. In R. B. Stuart (Ed.), *Behavioral self-management: Strategies and outcomes*. New York: Brunner/Mazel.

Bootzin, R. R., & Engle-Friedman, M. (1981). The assessment of insomnia. *Behavioral Assessment, 3*, 107–126.

Bootzin, R. R., Engle-Friedman, M., & Hazlewood, L. (1983). Insomnia. In P. M. Lewinsohn & L. Teri (Eds.), *Clinical geropsychology: New directions in assessment and treatment*. New York: Pergamon Press.

Bootzin, R. R., & Nicassio, P. (1978). Behavioral treatments for insomnia. In M. Hersen, R. M. Eisler, and P. M. Miller (Eds.), *Progress in behavior modification* (Vol. 6). New York: Academic Press.

Borkovec, T. D. (1982). Insomnia. *Journal of Consulting and Clinical Psychology, 50*, 880–895.

Espie, C. A., Lindsay, W. R., & Brooks, D. N. (1988). Substituting behavioural treatment for drugs in the treatment of insomnia: An exploratory study. *Journal of Behavior Therapy and Experimental Psychiatry, 19*, 51–56.

Espie, C. A., Lindsay, W. R., Brooks, D. N., Hood, E. M., & Turvey, T. (1989). A controlled comparative investigation of psychological treatments for chronic sleep-onset insomnia. *Behaviour Research and Therapy, 27*, 79–88.

Morin, C. M., & Azrin, H. N. (1987). Stimulus control and imagery training in treating sleep-maintenance insomnia. *Journal of Consulting and Clinical Psychology, 55*, 260–262.

CHAPTER THREE

Stimulus Control in a Group Setting

PATRICIA LACKS

INTRODUCTION

Stimulus control treatment for insomnia, originally developed by Richard Bootzin (1977), was designed to be applied to individuals. We used a small-group method of delivering this intervention. We chose this group approach strictly to conserve scarce research funds. However, after treating both groups and individuals, we became convinced that the group approach was the superior method of delivering these services.

The techniques reported in this chapter were developed over an eight-year period during which my colleague Amy Bertelson and I collaborated on a program of research, treating over 400 chronic insomniacs in seven treatment outcome studies (e.g., Lacks, Bertelson, Gans, & Kunkel, 1983). These were people who averaged at least 30 minutes of sleeplessness per night (mean = 77 minutes) for at least six months (mean duration = 13 years). They ranged in age from 18 to 78 years, were mostly female, white, well-educated, had a wide range in severity of sleep problems, and included clients with primary complaints of either sleep-onset or sleep-maintenance insomnia. Results have been very promising. For sleep-onset insomnia, average time to fall asleep was reduced from 72 minutes at baseline to 40 minutes after four weeks of treatment, 36 minutes at follow-up 6 to 12 weeks after intervention, and 30 minutes per night at a one-year follow-up. Comparable figures for sleep-maintenance insomnia were 88 minutes before treatment, 54 minutes posttreatment, and 46 and 44 minutes at the two follow-ups.

Patricia Lacks • Psychology Department, Washington University, St. Louis, Missouri 63130.

Using relatively stringent statistical criteria for clinical significance, 39 percent of these volunteers made a reliable change and 23 percent joined the ranks of good sleepers after only four weeks of treatment. By short-term follow-up, 47 percent showed real gains and 33 percent were good sleepers. Deterioration rates were less than 1 percent. By the one-year follow-up, 63 percent of the volunteers had at least a 50 percent decrease in the initial complaint and 31 percent reported that they "no longer have insomnia" (Lacks & Powlishta, 1989).

METHOD

Assessment of the Problem

Insomnia is not a specific disease but a complaint that can result from a number of factors, including organic sleep pathology (e.g., sleep apnea, nocturnal myoclonus, restless legs, or narcolepsy), painful medical conditions such as arthritis, physiological malfunction, use of hypnotic medications or other drugs, psychopathology such as depression or schizophrenia, emotional upset and stress, personality style such as rigid and compulsive, and learned behaviors. In order to choose the optimum treatment for this disorder, one must make a thorough assessment of the nature of the sleep disturbance and the source of the complaint (Association of Sleep Disorders Centers, 1979).

We always begin with a detailed personal history using a written 48-item Sleep History Questionnaire; if half the items are answered in the positive direction, they are to be followed up by oral interview questions. A more thorough but time-consuming approach is to conduct an interview such as the 53-item Structured Sleep History Interview (Lacks, 1987). These two instruments tap seven broad categories:

1. Description of the insomnia problem
2. Psychological contributing factors
3. Sleep hygiene
4. Psychopathology
5. Organic sleep disorders
6. Serious medical problems
7. Previous treatment of the insomnia

It is also helpful to question the client's bed partner to elicit history such as snoring, nighttime thrashing, and daytime sleepiness that may be helpful in making a diagnosis of organic sleep pathology.

To assess anxiety, tense and obsessive personality style, and psychopathology, especially depression, we administer the Minnesota Multiphasic Personality Inventory (MMPI) and, if depression is suspected, the Beck Depression Inventory (Beck, 1967). We try to discriminate between insomnia caused by depression and sleep disturbance that develops first and, over time, causes the person to feel hopeless, helpless, and demoralized. Specific measures of stress, anxiety, mood, and medical complaints may also be given.

An important component of our preliminary assessment is the Daily Sleep Diary (Lacks, 1987, 1988). It is used to monitor the subjective complaint of insomnia continuously from baseline through treatment and follow-up. The diary has four questions about sleep the previous night (minutes to fall asleep, times awakened in the night, length of each awake period, and total time slept) and six questions about the quality of sleep and daytime performance. A question about the use of sleep-inducing medication can be added. To ensure monitoring on a daily basis and reduce the possibility of retrospective estimates, our clients complete the diaries on pre-stamped forms upon awakening and mail them every day. Each client's progress can then be reviewed before the next treatment session. Because of large night-to-night variability of sleep, we use a two-week baseline period.

We also usually administer specialized measures of behaviors and attitudes associated with the sleep disturbance, such as awareness and practice of sleep hygiene principles (Lacks & Rotert, 1986), cognitive and somatic arousal (Nicassio, Mendlowitz, Fussell, & Petras, 1985), and self-efficacy or personal control over the sleep process (Lacks, 1987). Sleep hygiene includes the topics of caffeine, alcohol, and nicotine usage, exercise, sleep scheduling, prebedtime relaxation, and bedroom noise, light, and temperature.

A thorough assessment of any sleep complaint should include a physical history and medical examination. If it is suspected that a client has organic sleep pathology, a referral for polysomnography is in order. However, evaluation in a sleep laboratory is an expensive process, and not all communities have this kind of facility. The risk of an organic basis for a sleep disorder is higher in older adults and in those with complaints of sleep-maintenance problems or excessive daytime sleepiness. If a thorough evaluation, including an interview with the bed partner, reveals no evidence for organic sleep pathology, even in those at higher risk, a brief course of behavior therapy will be used, but with swift referral to a sleep disorders center if there is not quick response to treatment.

Clients believed to have organic sleep pathology, serious psychiatric disorders, substance abuse, or chronic pain are referred elsewhere for treatment. If the person appears to have an underlying psychiatric or medical basis for insomnia, treatment of the initial cause should always be undertaken first. However, if the person has suffered with insomnia for more than a few months, it is likely that maladaptive sleep behaviors are being maintained by conditioned factors and behavior therapy may be a valuable adjunct treatment.

Another pretreatment issue is whether or not to have the client discontinue the use of sleep-inducing medications. Our belief is that it is always preferable to do so because it is well established that hypnotics do alter patterns of sleep as well as result in a variety of side effects. Sometimes withdrawal alone from sleep medication is sufficient to eliminate the sleep disturbance. The clients are referred back to the prescribing physicians with the advice to withdraw gradually, lowering medication once or twice a week. Clients may need a good deal of support during this time. They may experience transient rebound insomnia for up to four weeks, depending on their medication, dosage, and length of usage. Clients are strongly warned of the rebound effect to avoid a rush back to their drugs (Kirmil-Gray, Eagleston, Thoresen, & Zarcone, 1985).

Elements of the Behavior Therapy

The therapist is a key element in this group therapy. The goal is to move the client from a passive, pill-taking mode to a problem-solving, self-reliant mode. To be successful, the therapist should be self-confident, knowledgeable about sleep and sleep disorders, experienced, organized, and optimistic. Of course, the therapist will have more chance of success if he or she has a sense of humor to lighten the proceedings and can rapidly develop rapport with the group members. Modeling self-disclosure, openness, and a problem-solving stance will also help.

The behavioral strategies of this treatment package are organized within a highly structured format of lessons, group discussion, and questions and answers. Group discussion must be controlled, guided, and always made to enhance, not detract from or become tangential to, the main purpose. The therapist must be a directive group leader or facilitator who gives regular feedback to clients, reinforces their efforts, and encourages further problem solving. The therapy can be accomplished in four or five sessions of about an hour each with 90 minutes for the first session.

In our experience, stimulus control treatment delivered in a group format yields results superior to those achieved by treating one person at a time. The primary advantage appears to be the element of accountability. The therapist of the individual client may be too understanding of lack of compliance with the sometimes difficult instructions of this treatment. In the group setting, however, the same nonadhering client meets with a more forceful reaction from the other group members who are less willing to tolerate noncompliance. Clients also report that it is important for them to meet other reasonable, seemingly normal people who have suffered for many years from poor sleep. They are relieved to know that they are not alone or "crazy" and that it is acceptable to seek help for such a problem. Participants also report that they benefit greatly from the chance to air their problems in a supportive atmosphere. With some help from the therapist, groups usually develop quick camaraderie, cohesion, and friendship.

Because this group process has proved to be so important to therapy in this target group, the therapist should promote it actively. If the therapist dominates the proceedings, is the source of all information and advice, the "expert" with the "correct" answers, the group members will say little. The setting will be more like a classroom with people taking notes and asking occasional questions. There will probably also be little improvement in sleep. The philosophy should be that when it comes to problem solving, six heads are better than one. It is going to be a collaborative effort; therefore, each person should plan to be actively involved. If any clients hang back, the therapist must actively help them to participate.

From our experience, the ideal group size is five to seven members. Having fewer members makes it more difficult to foster group process; more are harder to manage, and group members feel shortchanged of individual attention. We have also found it advantageous to have groups be homogeneous as to type of sleep problem. We have mixed men and women successfully, as well as younger and older adults. The inexperienced group therapist should read some additional material on the special issues of the group approach (Merritt & Walley, 1977).

Basic sleep education is another key element of this therapy. Many insomnia sufferers lack this knowledge and also have misconceptions about sleep. Therefore, the first session begins with a brief, basic overview of sleep, and additional information is given throughout subsequent sessions. Included is information about the prevalence of insomnia, the myth of the necessity of eight hours of sleep for everyone, that waking up several times in the night for brief periods is normal, that loss of sleep does not lead to as dire consequences as they believe, and that there can be a behavioral basis for the development of persistent sleep troubles (American Medical Association, 1984; Hauri, 1982).

Other important elements of this therapy are the process of daily self-monitoring, which helps the client adopt the role of "personal scientist," promotion of a sense of self-control to reduce the feeling of helplessness and increase knowledge of concrete and specific solutions, and instructions in sleep hygiene and sleep scheduling. For the latter, clients are required to have a regular awakening time each day and to eliminate naps. Eventually they will become drowsy at about the same time each night.

Of course, the chief feature of the intervention to be described will be the stimulus control instructions themselves. Clients are taught concrete ways to reassociate the bed and bedroom with rapid sleep onset by curtailing all sleep-incompatible behaviors in the bedroom that serve as cues for staying awake.

FOUR GROUP TREATMENT SESSIONS

Session 1

The therapist begins by "breaking the ice"—sharing personal, clinical, or research experiences with insomnia and briefly relating the research support for behavior therapy for sleep disturbance. Next, the group members introduce themselves, briefly describing their own sleep problems, while the therapist fosters the beginning of group interaction. The therapist begins by giving some kind of specific information and then turns to the group members for reactions, personal examples, questions, discussion, and suggestions.

The first focus of this session is defining the principle of stimulus control, applying it to sleep difficulties, and briefly describing the stimulus control treatment that will follow. Participants are told that they will also receive education about sleep, will be told the rules for good sleep hygiene, and will learn to monitor their own sleep. The therapist emphasizes consistency of practice to learn new, permanent sleep habits and stresses that these changes will take a full four sessions to accomplish.

At this point, a copy of the nine "Sleep Hygiene Rules" (see Table 1) is handed out. After the clients read the list, the therapist goes over each point, providing further explanation. Each rule is read and elaborated upon. Each client then discusses his or her current behavior for it and elicits *concrete strategies* for how he or she will implement the rule. The therapist always makes a record of these planned strategies so that they can be checked in future sessions.

As an example, for rule 1, the therapist explains that many insomnia sufferers go to bed before they are sleepy, thinking that if they give themselves 10 to 12 hours in bed they may be able to get eight hours of sleep. But if they are not drowsy, they may toss and turn, begin to think, and become mentally and physically aroused. Being tired does not necessarily mean readiness for sleep. Discussion will center around how clients are now determining when they will go to bed (e.g., fixed or flexible bedtime or linked to spouse's bedtime) and how they feel when they go to bed. Many poor sleepers have to be concretely taught to recognize the cues of drowsiness (e.g., yawning, rubbing eyes, flickering eyelids).

Table 1. Sleep Hygiene Rules[a]

1. Do not go to bed until you are drowsy.
2. Get up at approximately the same time each morning, including weekends. If you feel you must get up later on weekends, allow yourself a maximum of one hour later arising.
3. Do not take naps.

These first three rules will give you a consistent sleep rhythm and synchronize your biological clock. With time, your bedtime, or the time you become drowsy, will also tend to become regularized.

4. Do not drink alcohol later than two hours prior to bedtime.
5. Do not consume caffeine after about 4 P.M., or within six hours prior to bedtime. Learn all the foods, beverages, and medications that contain caffeine.
6. Do not smoke within several hours prior to your bedtime.
7. Exercise regularly. The best time to exercise is in the late afternoon. Avoid strenuous physical exertion after 6 P.M.
8. Use common sense to make your sleep environment most conducive to sleep. Arrange for a comfortable temperature and minimum levels of sound, light, and noise.
9. If you are accustomed to it, have a light carbohydrate or dairy snack before bedtime (e.g., crackers, graham crackers, milk, or cheese). Do not eat chocolate or large amounts of sugar. Avoid excessive fluids. If you awaken in the middle of the night, do not have a snack then or you may find that you begin to wake up habitually at that time feeling hungry.

[a] From Lacks (1987). Copyright 1987 Pergamon Press, Inc. Reprinted by permission of Pergamon Press, Inc.

For rule 4, the therapist explains that alcohol is a depressant that, if timed accurately, may help a person relax and fall asleep. However, it leads to restless, nonrestorative sleep, and the tendency to wake up during the night. As part of rule 5, it is explained that caffeine is a powerful, long-lasting stimulant that interferes with the natural sleep cycle. Many myths abound in this area, and clients are surprisingly ignorant of what substances contain caffeine and in what amounts. Clients are asked to make sure that all their medications and over-the-counter preparations contain no stimulants. Often, medications can be taken earlier in the day or substitutes without stimulants can be prescribed. Further details of how sleep hygiene instruction is handled can be found in *Behavioral Treatment for Persistent Insomnia* (Lacks, 1987).

The therapist now passes out a separate sheet of Stimulus Control Instructions (see Table 2). Instruction 1 lists activities that are a "misuse" of the bed and bedroom and encourage wakefulness. These activities include eating, talking on the telephone, lying awake, thinking, worrying, and feeling frustrated about not falling asleep. If the bed is reserved solely for sleep, then climbing into bed will be a strong cue for the client to fall asleep. Clients discuss other activities they currently do in bed. They are helped to find other places and other times to engage in these activities. For example,

Table 2. Stimulus Control Instructions[a]

1. Do not use your bed or bedroom for any activity other than sleep. You should not watch television, read, talk on the telephone, worry, argue with your spouse, or eat in bed. The only exception to this rule is that you may engage in sexual activity in bed.
2. Establish a set of regular presleep routines to signal that bedtime approaches. Lock the door, plug in the coffee machine, brush teeth, set the alarm, and perform any other behaviors that make sense for this time of night. Do these activities in the same order each night. Use your preferred sleep posture and combination of favorite pillows and blankets.
3. When you get into bed, turn out the lights with the intention of going right to sleep. If you cannot fall asleep within a short time (about ten minutes), get up and go into another room. Engage in some quiet activity until you begin to feel drowsy and then return to the bedroom to sleep.
4. If you still do not fall asleep within a brief time, repeat the previous step. Repeat this process as often as it is necessary throughout the night. Use this same procedure if you awaken in the middle of the night and do not return to sleep within about ten minutes.

[a]From Lacks (1987). Copyright 1987 Pergamon Press, Inc. Reprinted by permission of Pergamon Press, Inc.

it is appropriate to plan the next day's schedule and set out clothes and materials for it. This should be done earlier in the evening and outside the bedroom as much as possible. Clients again offer concrete suggestions for themselves and other group members. Often, these plans will include moving things such as television sets and desks out of the bedroom. Again, the therapist notes these plans for reference during future sessions.

Instruction 2 outlines how a set of regular presleep routines can serve as a signal of the approach of bedtime and can promote a feeling of drowsiness. The hour before bedtime should be one of preparing for sleep, a time to wind down. This should be an hour of relaxation (e.g., warm bath, reading, watching television), of putting aside the troubles of the past day and of the coming day. Activities that are arousing (e.g., exercise, phone calls, planning) should be scheduled for earlier in the day. More specific strategies on this point are covered in session 2.

Instructions 3 and 4 are the most essential part of stimulus control treatment for insomnia, the most difficult for clients to implement, and the ones they will most resist. Because the object is to connect the bed and bedroom with sleeping, it is undesirable for them to lie awake in bed for long periods, feeling frustrated. Then the bed becomes a signal for thinking, tossing and turning, and worrying and becoming anxious about insomnia. As a result, the insomnia sufferer often comes to fight the bed or even comes to see the bed as the *enemy*.

Discussion of these two instructions will be lively, filled with clients' reasons why they cannot possibly get out of bed during the night: it will wake them more fully and make sleep more difficult, it will disturb their spouse's sleep, it is too cold, and many others. All of these difficulties can be addressed. The therapist must never budge in the conviction that these two principles are the core of the treatment and must take an active problem-solving approach to their objections. First the group and then the therapist comes up with concrete suggestions for implementing these two rules. Each person is helped to make a well-thought-out plan for compliance. For example, if the person chooses to read when getting out of bed, he or she should select the appropriate reading material, and set it out along with a robe, slippers, reading glasses, and a flashlight. He or she should choose a location to read and have that spot arranged to facilitate the nighttime activity.

Good sleepers take 10 to 20 minutes to fall asleep. Clients will need to leave the bed after about ten minutes of sleeplessness (but they should not be watching the clock) both at the beginning of the night and later, if they awaken in the night.

It is important for the therapist to emphasize how difficult this aspect of the treatment will be, as any new behaviors are. Clients should expect sleep to get worse the first week before gradually improving. The therapist should warn them that they may feel that the treatment is worse than the original sleep problem they came with. The therapist predicts that they will be getting up many times during the first few nights, that they will feel tired and have impaired daytime functioning, and that they may consider dropping out of the treatment program. But the situation is only temporary, and if they persist, they should meet with success.

The last few minutes of each session are reserved for assigning homework to extend the treatment into each day rather than just the hour session per week. The homework consists mainly of close monitoring and charting sleep-related behaviors to identify and strengthen the cues associated with falling asleep quickly. Clients also need to identify and weaken those cues associated with staying awake. The therapist reemphasizes that the Daily Sleep Diary is an important part of the homework. Another monitoring form, the Practice Record (Lacks, 1987), is a set of six questions on a chart that includes the seven days of the week. Each day, clients indicate degree of drowsiness upon retiring the night before, what time they got up that morning, activities from dinner to bedtime, activities while getting ready for bed, any activities carried out in bed, and thoughts while in bed. Clients are told that much of the time in future sessions will be devoted to reviewing these practice records and suggesting solutions for problems, so they must fill out the records faithfully and bring them to all sessions. They are also given a chart of Times Out of Bed (number of times out of bed for each night of the treatment) to fill in each morning. All these forms promote compliance with the treatment, provide information to the therapist and client, and show the treatment progress. They are essential to the treatment and not just data for research.

Subsequent Sessions

The major part of the next three sessions will be spent in collaborative troubleshooting of any difficulties that clients have encountered during the week in adhering to the treatment. Some new material will be introduced in each of these subsequent sessions; however, the problem solving will take most of the time. We have developed a standard ten-point format for the therapist to use for this process:

1. Review the Practice Records before the session begins to determine if there have been problems with adherence during the week. You will then be prepared to anticipate the general content of the session and to combat client exaggerations of lack of progress. As the session begins, return the forms to the clients and, for each of the six homework questions, go around the group asking all members to report their experiences and difficulties. After the session, retain the homework for future reference or planning.

2. Get a precise description for every problem reported during the week. Was the problem due to inability or unwillingness to implement the procedures, or did the environment make adherence difficult?

3. Elicit group solutions to the problem. For each suggestion, encourage discussion and sharing of experiences. What worked for other clients in similar circumstances? Generate as many solutions as possible without criticism, then combine and improve suggestions, making them as specific as possible.

4. Always stay committed to the stimulus control approach. Emphasize the importance of following the rules every night. Do not tolerate any breaking of treatment rules or not following through on previous suggestions. Remind clients of the treatment rationale and its proven effectiveness.

5. Decide on a course of action for the coming week. Choose the most useful solution, the one most likely to be implemented. Communicate confidence to the client that problems are common, routine, and solvable. Predict any likely side effects of the planned action.

6. Instruct the client to experiment with the behavior during the week. Stress a "personal scientist" strategy for problem solving that includes trial and error, keeping records, and fine tuning.

7. If no solution is evident, defer action while the client carefully monitors the problem for another week. During the week, try to devise a solution.

8. Always follow up on progress made during the week on problems discussed during the previous sessions. This action will convey that you are always monitoring client progress and you take adherence to treatment seriously. Find new solutions if necessary.

9. Restate the point that significant improvement will take the full four weeks. Clients are learning new habits and these behaviors must be practiced consistently over time to work and become routine. Respond to lack of change with encouragement and patience.

10. Give plenty of praise and encouragement, especially for following the rules and new routines. Use the group members to praise and support each other.

Session 2

The therapist should expect this session to be the hardest. Many participants will feel frustrated, discouraged, tired, and angry that their symptoms worsened during this week. The therapist should remind them that this was the predicted outcome. If their sleep did deteriorate during the first week, then they are right on course and following the treatment instructions. Therapy is taking its expected path.

The dominant topic will be the extreme aversion clients have to getting out of bed after ten minutes of sleeplessness. They will report multiple reasons why this is an unreasonable request. Even if tempted to remove or soften this requirement, the therapist must not do it! Instead, everyone's efforts are focused on finding ways to make it less aversive. The short-term discomfort is contrasted with the long-term satisfaction of improved sleep that will make leaving the bed no longer necessary. Usually at least one group member has been very compliant and is already beginning to notice improvement. The therapist uses this member as a model and someone to encourage or coach the others. If disturbing the bed partner is given as a reason for not leaving the bed, the client is encouraged to discuss this problem with the bed partner. Most bedmates are willing to cooperate and tolerate some temporary inconvenience to help the client gain improved sleep. Clients also often report difficulty adhering to sleep hygiene rules, especially giving up substances or long-standing practices that result in strong feelings of deprivation. Other typical concerns are kinds of activities to engage in while waiting to become drowsy, how to estimate the ten-minute period in bed, and cues to know when clients are drowsy.

The designated new material for this session is establishment of a set of prebed routines. These routines will eventually cue the client to become sleepy and ready for bed. The therapist has the group review their homework forms and look for patterns in their before-bed activities. These are used as a starting point to develop a routine. Each client constructs a list of the behaviors he or she wants to make routine and places them in a logical and convenient order. The therapist makes sure none of the activities are mentally arousing; those that are should be rescheduled for earlier in the evening. The therapist and the clients should then each have a written record of the planned routine that will be carried out in the same order each night right after the client begins to feel sleepy. The therapist ends the session by reminding clients to keep filling out the three homework forms.

Session 3

As in Session 2, the first half of this meeting will be spent reviewing the Practice Records in detail and troubleshooting any problems. The therapist should always refer to the notes made of planned behaviors and check on clients' success in carrying out their individual assignments. The therapist reviews each person's progress with his or her presleep routine and makes modifications where necessary

The new material for this session deals with discovering personal behaviors associated with good and poor sleep. By reviewing practice records and group discussion, the therapist generates for each client a list of behaviors that have positive effects on sleep and those that have negative effects. Examples of the latter could be having evening coffee or a slice of chocolate cake, worrying, reading certain kinds of materials, and discussing certain topics. Positive effects might follow daytime exercise, an hour of prebedtime relaxation, or pleasant evening conversation with a spouse. The therapist encourages clients to examine their own records, comparing nights of adequate sleep to those where their sleep was disturbed. The therapist discusses ways to avoid the disturbing activities and to make the enhancing behaviors a part of the daily routine. The session ends with the usual homework of the three monitoring forms and continued work on behaviors that promote good and poor sleep.

Session 4

In addition to the regular troubleshooting, there are two new topics for this final session. First, it is time for the therapist to express the positive expectation that clients should not begin to see the fruits of their efforts. Second are instructions to continue faithfully the new behaviors so that the clients will experience continued improvement and can cement these new habits to maintain their gains. After the coming week they may choose to phase out the self-monitoring. It is explained how to prevent an occasional bad night from developing into a pattern of insomnia. The therapist gives special encouragement for continued work to those clients who have not shown progress, explaining that they may need more than four weeks of effort.

ADDITIONAL TREATMENT ISSUES

Predictors of Outcome

In our investigations, we found five factors that made a contribution to sleep improvement. A better response was found with clients who were younger, had a later age of onset of insomnia, had a longer duration of the current problem, showed less psychopathology on the MMPI, and received stimulus control therapy rather than some other type (Lacks & Powlishta, 1989). To illustrate, let us look at a group of 109 clients at the end of four weeks of treatment for sleep-onset insomnia. Those who had 0-1 MMPI scales in the pathological range (T-Score > 70) showed a 56 percent decrease in their time to fall asleep, those with 2-4 pathological scales showed a 41 percent decrease, and those with 5-6 scales only a 7 percent decrease. Of the same group of 109 participants, those who received stimulus control showed a 58 percent decrease of complaint at posttreatment, while those who received other treatments showed a 37 percent improvement rate. By short-term follow-up (one to three months posttreatment), none of these factors any longer predicted amount of improvement.

Informally, we have collected examples of difficult clients and situations that occur regularly. Probably the most frequent problem that interferes with progress is client resistance to following treatment instructions. Examples of this resistance are not trying the suggestions while insisting they will not work, persistently playing the devil's advocate or "yes, but . . ." with the therapist, complaining that the treatment received is not what was expected or desired, claiming to be diligently adhering to treatment although the therapist is doubtful, and talking at length about tangential issues. Typical unrelated topics are dream analysis, folk remedies (e.g., warm milk, calcium, vitamins), types of mattresses, and magical or easy solutions to sleep problems. We have also seen clients who want to talk at length about seemingly peripheral personal problems (e.g., marital or job unhappiness) that they insist are involved in their sleep disturbances. A few clients may even introduce bizarre, disturbing topics that the therapist may have to discourage in a brief, private meeting.

We have one basic response to these situations that threaten the outcome: we are trying to provide a specific treatment for insomnia that has well-established efficacy, in contrast to many other remedies that clients may know about. We are trying to provide this treatment within a limited time to conserve costs and time. To be effective, we must cover all the planned material in four brief sessions. Therefore, we do not want the group to become sidetracked on topics that are not part of this specific regimen. We also emphasize that most of the group members have suffered from insomnia for a considerable length of time and have little to lose by participating fully, trying all suggestions for the very short time of four weeks. Even if some aspects of the therapy are burdensome, they are designed to alleviate the discomfort of chronic insomnia. We remind clients that, in our experience, adherence to the total treatment package usually leads to improvement, while nonadherence is almost guaranteed to result in no change or even a worsening of sleep. Many clients have been able to reverse the deleterious effects of 20 to 30 years of insomnia with only four weeks of hard work.

Another problem client is one who dominates the proceedings by continuously talking, interrupting, and bullying other group members. This person does not really seem interested in making changes in his or her own life. Because this type of client has limited self-control, the therapist will have to assertively provide that control in the group. The silent client, while less threatening to the group progress, is unlikely to make personal progress. The therapist pushes this client to participate by regularly calling on him or her, asking for details even if the person insists that everything is going well.

In general, clients who have many physical complaints, who whine, who have such performance anxiety that they will not try anything that might worsen sleep even temporarily, who are rigid, demanding, closed to new ideas, and insist that nothing will work have a poor prognosis for change. In contrast, those who are flexible, open to new ideas, cooperative, psychologically healthy, and are willing to think in terms of long-term goals have an excellent prognosis. The latter group can usually be identified early in treatment, and they are called on often in group sessions to help with the former group of clients. They are often effective at countering the arguments of the less cooperative clients.

Alterations for the Sleep Maintenance Client

Most of this chapter has focused on the person who has sleep-onset insomnia, or difficulty getting to sleep. For those who wake in the middle of the night and have trouble returning to sleep, these same methods can be used with slight alterations (Morin & Azrin, 1987). It appears that many of the same sleep-interfering behaviors also take place during the middle of the night. The therapist will have to change language, using phrases like "in the middle of the night" instead of "when you go to bed" and "remain asleep" instead of "fall asleep." Parallel changes can be made on the homework forms. It is normal to wake up several times during the night. It is a problem only if you do not fall back asleep quickly. This fact helps clients who have developed performance anxiety because they think any awakening reflects insomnia. It must be remembered that many poor sleepers suffer from both types of insomnia, but most of them can tell which problem is primary for them; they should be placed in a treatment group designed for that primary problem. In our research, we have found stimulus control equally effective with both types of sleep disturbance (Lacks, Bertelson, Sugerman, & Kunkel, 1983).

The Older Adult

Many clinicians hold stereotyped attitudes that older adults are rigid, unenergetic, and unable to learn new behaviors. Their psychological problems are often seen as a normal part of old age or due to irreversible organic brain disorders. Consequently, these older clients are more often treated with medication. In contrast to these beliefs, we have had very positive experiences in treating the sleep problems of older adults with behavior therapy (e.g., Puder, Lacks, Bertelson, & Storandt, 1983). These results are encouraging because sleep disturbance increases with age, and behavior therapy is a much safer intervention for them than hypnotic medications. At this time, our success has been confined to older adults, up to age 78, who are independent, self-sufficient, and relatively well educated.

There are some special considerations for working with older adults, just as there are some realistic ways in which they differ from younger clients. Many have had some sensory loss, such as impaired vision or hearing, which they may not reveal to the therapist. It is wise in working with this older group for the therapist to take certain precautions: reduce background noise, speak in the lowest vocal range while facing the client, have bright overhead lighting and clear handouts. Also, the therapist should expect to have poor attendance during bad weather because older clients have a very strong fear of falling on ice or becoming ill from cold temperatures. The therapist working with the older adult will also have to be familiar with and empathetic to the special developmental issues of this age group: bereavement, retirement, dying, decreased personal autonomy, loneliness, feeling insecure in their home at night, and encroaching disability. There are also some realistic health problems in this age group that can interfere with sleep. Sensitivity to caffeine, noise, and temperature increases with age. Gastric reflux may require avoiding evening food and propping up the mattress. Diuretics for hypertension may cause frequent nighttime awakenings unless evening fluids are curtailed.

Many sleep researchers believe that the most important factor in improving older adult sleep is regulation of the circadian rhythm (Bootzin, Engle-Friedman, & Hazelwood, 1983; Miles & Dement, 1980). The best method for anchoring the sleep–wake schedule is to have the client get up at the same time every morning regardless of when he or she went to bed or how much sleep was obtained. Many older insomnia sufferers spend 10 to 12 hours in bed each night trying to get adequate sleep or because they do not have any pressing reason to get out of bed. Encouragement to develop regular daytime schedules that include socialization, activities, and physical exercise will aid regularization of sleep rhythm and will promote an active, less sedentary, stimulating life that will serve to enhance sleep.

We have successfully treated the insomnia of older persons, both in groups made up solely of older adults and in groups of mixed ages. However, some older people learn more slowly and the treatment may have to be lengthened slightly and proceed more slowly for them. The therapist may have to be more patient and provide more repetition, clarification, and support.

DISCUSSION

We have had considerable success in improving the sleep of participants who have been predominantly female, white, middle-class, and well educated. These are the individuals who are likely to want a nondrug solution that promotes self-responsibility and self-control. A less educated, clinic population may not do as well with these techniques. Our clients were also well screened to eliminate most cases of depression and other serious psychiatric disorders, physical illness, and chronic pain. Because these conditions are known to disrupt sleep (e.g., 44 percent of all psychotropic drug prescriptions in five major oncology centers were for disturbed sleep), it makes sense to look at the usefulness of behavioral treatment for insomnia in these groups. A few small studies using cancer patients have shown some initial success in improving sleep with behavior therapy (Cannici, Malcolm, & Peek, 1983).

Although we believe that we have had good success, only a third of our clients have become good sleepers and about half have experienced significant reduction of their original complaints. Insomnia is a complex problem that affects different people in different ways and has a multitude of causes. Therefore, there are probably many poor sleepers for whom no single remedy will provide sufficient relief. One possible approach to increasing effectiveness may be to individualize methods more or to provide more than one treatment.

Other chapters in this book will present these types of approach, including integration of stimulus control with other methods. However, clinicians will need to be cautious in their efforts to combine treatments. Some methods may work against each other. Also, some researchers have found multiple-component treatments to be less effective than single-component approaches (Turner, DiTomasso, & Giles, 1982). One thought is that each component may need a certain amount of time to be learned and incorporated into a behavioral routine. If clients are asked to learn too many skills at one time, it may defeat the purpose.

As a solution to these difficulties, we have proposed a treatment model based on the concept of "successive sieves." In this strategy, each client first receives the standard stimulus control treatment package that includes sleep hygiene instructions. Because this package has shown the best research results and because it is brief and easier to learn than other approaches, it seems sensible to begin with it. This four-week treatment should be followed by a four-week consolidation phase where practice of the new skills is encouraged. After this first phase, all participants who have not achieved good sleeper status would be given a second, individualized, symptom-specific treatment for four weeks, again followed by a practice period. If necessary, even a third phase could be added. Treatments that could be used in subsequent phases include autogenic training, sleep restriction, progressive relaxation, or some form of cognitive refocusing. The latter may be especially useful because the majority of poor sleepers complain of nighttime cognitive arousal.

Patricia Lacks received her Ph.D. in clinical psychology in 1966 and since 1972 has been a faculty member in the Department of Psychology at Washington University in St. Louis, Missouri. She is also in part-time private practice as a clinical psychologist with a cognitive/behavioral orientation. Dr. Lacks has been active in insomnia treatment outcome research since 1980 and has published and delivered a number of papers on these findings. Her book *Behavioral Treatment for Persistent Insomnia* was published in 1987. She has also published papers on psychological assessment and the 1984 book *Bender Gestalt Screening for Brain Dysfunction*.

RECOMMENDED READINGS

American Medical Association. (1984). *Guide to better sleep*. New York: Random House.

This book is an excellent self-help guide that includes basic sleep education, sleep hygiene, and concrete suggestions for improving sleep.

Association of Sleep Disorders Centers. (1979). Diagnostic classification of sleep and arousal disorders. *Sleep, 2,* 1–137.

This reference describes in detail the criteria for making a diagnosis of sleep disturbance. The widely accepted diagnostic criteria include four major categories of sleep disturbance each with a number of subtypes.

Bootzin, R. R. (1977). Effects of self-control procedures for insomnia. In R. Stuart (Ed.), *Behavioral self-management: Strategies, techniques, and outcome.* New York: Brunner/Mazel, pp. 176–195.

This article provides additional details about stimulus control treatment for insomnia.

Lacks, P. (1987). *Behavioral treatment for persistent insomnia.* New York: Pergamon Press.

This book has additional information about various types of sleep disturbance and details of the treatment procedures presented in this chapter. It also contains basic facts about normal sleep.

REFERENCES

American Medical Association. (1984). *Guide to better sleep.* New York: Random House.

Association of Sleep Disorders Centers. (1979). Diagnostic classification of sleep and arousal disorders. *Sleep, 2,* 1–137.

Beck, A. T. (1967). *Depression: Clinical, experimental, and theoretical aspects.* New York: Harper & Row.

Bootzin, R. R. (1977). Effects of self-control procedures for insomnia. In R. Stuart (Ed.), *Behavioral self-management: Strategies, techniques, and outcome.* New York: Brunner/Mazel, pp. 179–195.

Bootzin, R. R., Engle-Friedman, M., & Hazelwood, L. (1983). Insomnia. In P. M. Lewinsohn & L. Teri (Eds.), *Clinical geropsychology: New directions in assessment and treatment.* New York: Pergamon Press, pp. 81–115.

Cannici, J., Malcolm, R., & Peek, L. A. (1983). Treatment of insomnia in cancer patients using muscle relaxation training. *Journal of Behavior Therapy and Experimental Psychiatry, 14,* 251–256.

Hauri, P. (1982). *The sleep disorders.* Kalamazoo, MI: Upjohn.

Kirmil-Gray, K., Eagleston, J. R., Thoresen, C. E., & Zarcone, V. P. (1985). Brief consultation and stress management treatments for drug-dependent insomnia: Effects on sleep quality, self-efficacy, and daytime stress. *Journal of Behavioral Medicine, 8,* 79–99.

Lacks, P. (1987). *Behavioral treatment for persistent insomnia.* Elmsford, NY: Pergamon Press.

Lacks, P. (1988). Daily sleep dairy. In M. Hersen & A. S. Bellack (Eds.), *Dictionary of behavioral assessment techniques.* Elmsford, NY: Pergamon Press.

Lacks, P., Bertelson, A. D., Gans, L., & Kunkel, J. (1983). The effectiveness of three behavioral treatments for different degrees of sleep onset insomnia. *Behavior Therapy, 14,* 593–605.

Lacks, P., Bertelson, A. D., Sugerman, J. L., & Kunkel, J. (1983). The treatment of sleep maintenance insomnia with stimulus control techniques. *Behaviour Research and Therapy, 21,* 291–295.

Lacks, P., & Powlishta, K. (1989). Improvement following behavioral treatment for insomnia: Clinical significance, long-term maintenance, and predictors of outcome. *Behavior Therapy, 20,* 117–134.

Lacks, P., & Rotert, M. (1986). Knowledge and practice of sleep hygiene techniques in insomniacs and good sleepers. *Behaviour Research and Therapy, 24,* 365–368.

Merritt, R. E., & Walley, D. D. (1977). *The group leader's handbook.* Champaign, IL: Research Press.

Miles, L. E., & Dement, W. C. (1980). Sleep and aging. *Sleep, 3,* 119–220.

Morin, C. M., & Azrin, N. H. (1987). Stimulus control and imagery training in treating sleep-maintenance insomnia. *Journal of Consulting and Clinical Psychology, 55,* 260–262.

Nicassio, P. M., Mendlowitz, D. R., Fussell, J. J., & Petras, L. (1985). The phenomenology of the pre-sleep state: The development of the Pre-sleep Arousal Scale. *Behaviour Research and Therapy, 23,* 263–271.

Puder, R., Lacks, P., Bertelson, A. D., & Storandt, M. (1983). Short-term stimulus control treatment of insomnia in older adults. *Behavior Therapy, 14,* 424–429.

Turner, R. M., DiTomasso, R., & Giles, T. (1982). Failures in the treatment of insomnia: A plea for differential diagnosis. In E. B. Foa (Ed.), *Failures in behavior therapy.* New York: Wiley, pp. 284–304.

CHAPTER FOUR

Sleep Restriction Therapy

PAUL B. GLOVINSKY AND ARTHUR J. SPIELMAN

INTRODUCTION

Drawing on clinical experience in sleep disorder centers and laboratory-based investigations, we are continuing to develop conceptual models as well as behavioral treatment strategies for insomnia. The technique reported on here, sleep restriction therapy, has had its effectiveness confirmed in laboratory and clinical studies and is now widely used in sleep disorders centers (Spielman, Saskin, & Thorpy, 1987; Friedman, Bliwise, Yesavage, & Salom, 1991; Morin, Kowatch, & Wade, 1989; Morin, Kowatch, & O'Shanick, 1990; Rubinstein, Rothenberg, Maheswaran, Tsai, Zozula, & Spielman, 1990).

Numerous classic studies conducted with noncomplaining subjects have shown that sleep becomes "robust" as a result of deprivation (Webb & Agnew, 1965, 1974). Subjects fall asleep more readily, sleep more deeply, have fewer awakenings, and easily maintain sleep until a wakeup call. These consequences of sleep deprivation are just what the insomniac hopes for. However, sleep deprivation also produces daytime sleepiness. Sleep restriction therapy was designed to exploit the consequences of sleep loss for enhancing nocturnal sleep while temporarily accepting daytime sleepiness as a side effect.

Paul B. Glovinsky and Arthur J. Spielman • Department of Psychology, The City College of the City University of New York, New York, New York and Insomnia Treatment Center, New York, New York 10017.

ASSESSMENT

The evaluation and treatment of a patient with insomnia covers many domains (Spielman, 1986; Spielman, Caruso, & Glovinsky, 1987). Here, we limit our discussion to issues that bear on the recommendation and conduct of sleep restriction therapy. Before our initial consultation, we ask the patient to fill out a medical history questionnaire and a two-week sleep diary. Using this information as well as that elicited during the clinical interview, we decide whether or not sleep restriction therapy is an appropriate first course of action. Although a diagnostic all-night polysomnographic recording has been shown to uncover potentially useful information, especially with older patients, its routine use is still a matter of debate (Edinger, Hoelscher, Webb, Marsh, Radtke, & Erwin, 1989). A recent meeting of experts at Stanford University concluded that recording all insomniacs prior to treatment was not practical and that, in the majority of cases, a behavioral approach to treatment was a rational first step. In older patients and when an insomnia proves intractable to treatment, a diagnostic sleep recording should be considered.

The sleep log yields subjective data concerning the duration, timing, and variability of sleep episodes. It also records whether or not the patient is in bed awake for lengthy stretches, for example, watching the late-night news or lolling about after the alarm clock has gone off in the morning. The clinical interview yields broader-scale information that is not only subjective, but also subject to more "editing" on the part of the patient. Thus, it is fairly common for a patient to report on interview that he or she naps or drinks coffee in the evening on only rare occasions yet produce a two-week sleep log with several such instances.

While a sleep log might yield more accurate numerical data, it cannot begin to convey the idiosyncracies of the patient's subjective experience of insomnia. Whether the bedroom is perceived as a haven or a prison or whether the patient's sense of physical and psychological vulnerability has been heightened by chronic sleep disturbances are issues that do not directly pertain to the administration of sleep restriction therapy. Yet they must ultimately be addressed if treatment is to succeed.

Sleep restriction therapy is generally effective in treating the most common forms of insomnia. Good responses can be obtained in patients complaining of difficulty falling and/or staying asleep, as well as in patients complaining of poor-quality sleep. The treatment is indicated in cases of chronic insomnia, with poor sleep recurring at least twice a week. It has worked best in those patients who report an hour or more of wakefulness over the course of their time in bed or highly fragmented sleep.

Sleep restriction therapy is inappropriate in the following instances: major affective disorder, sleep apnea, delayed sleep phase syndrome, and sleep disturbance due to "workshift" changes. These conditions are handled more effectively by other approaches. Because of the sleepiness produced initially, sleep restriction therapy should be deferred when important assignments are due at work and other occasions when full alertness is desired. It should also be deferred in favor of stimulus control instructions (Bootzin & Nicassio, 1978) when the history suggests that maladaptive conditioning plays an important role.

METHOD

Proper administration of sleep restriction therapy depends on the availability of a completed sleep log. On the basis of the sleep log, patients are assigned bedtime hours as follows. Total time in bed is set equal to the patient's estimate of how much he or she sleeps on average. In no case will we set time in bed below 4.5 hours. Time of arising from bed is set to the time when the patient generally awakens, and time of retiring is calculated accordingly. These appointed times yield a window for sleep. No napping is permitted outside this window. A detailed account of sleep restriction therapy has been presented elsewhere (Spielman, Saskin, & Thorpy, 1987).

Patients often ask if they have to be in bed trying to sleep during the scheduled bedtime. We do not insist on this. Patients may stay out late over the weekend, but they are still required to be out of bed in the morning at the designated time. We make it clear that the major import of the schedule is that they are to be neither in bed nor sleeping between the arising time and the retiring time. Furthermore, lying down outside of the scheduled bedtimes is not permitted.

In the original sleep restriction therapy procedure, adjustments to the initial sleep schedule (through alterations of retiring time) were made according to the following formula:

1. Increase by 15 minutes if the mean subjective sleep efficiency (sleep time/time in bed × 100 percent) over five nights was ≥ 90 percent.
2. Decrease by 15 minutes if the mean subjective sleep efficiency (sleep time/time in bed × 100 percent) over five nights was < 85 percent.

A number of modifications have been introduced in the course of refining this procedure:

1. In applying sleep restriction therapy to an elderly population, we lowered the sleep efficiency criteria by five percent to reflect ontogenetic changes in sleep continuity.

2. In practice, we found that patient compliance was enhanced if a relatively drastic initial reduction in time in bed was followed exclusively by increases in bedtime. We now rarely resort to curtailing bedtime beyond the initial reduction.
3. In that subgroup of patients who report little or no sleep no matter what objective measures may indicate, we have found that sleep restriction therapy must be modified; these patients never report high sleep efficiencies. For these patients, we instituted programmed increases in time in bed on a weekly basis (Rubinstein et al., 1990). The initial time in bed is determined according to subjective report; increases are scheduled that bring their bedtime up to seven hours. Further modifications are based on reported daytime performance, mood, and alertness.

Patients will respond much more favorably if they are prepared for sleep restriction therapy. Telling patients that the first two or three weeks of treatment are most difficult and that most patients complete the treatment in about 8 weeks informs them that they must give this treatment time to work. We stress that sleep changes slowly; a good or bad night or two is not our focus. We evaluate long-term trends because the treatment is designed to create robust sleep for the long haul, not yield a quick fix. In fact, over the short run, a host of daytime problems secondary to inadequate sleep is to be expected.

The probability of daytime sleepiness at the start of treatment should be stressed. In particular, drowsiness in the midafternoon and during the evening hours may present difficulty. It is crucial for the patient to have a plan ready for dealing with drowsiness; the initial prescribed bedtime is hours later than usual, fewer people are awake, stores are likely to be closed, and television programming may be uninteresting or soporific.

The patient should not be left to cast about for ways to keep busy and stay awake, but rather have a number of tasks at hand that are not mentally demanding or excessively stimulating. In the afternoon, exercise would be appropriate; in the evening, nonsedentary activities, such as light housekeeping, organizing a closet, putting photographs in a picture album, or record filing, will preclude inadvertent sleep episodes.

If the patient falls asleep in the late evening, no matter how briefly, that night's sleep may be a disaster. Also to be avoided are prolonged periods of listlessness. To bring this message home, we supply patients with a metaphor. They are asked to view the evening's activities and the preparations for bed as if they were piloting a glider in for a landing. If they lose altitude (get sleepy) too soon, they will land (fall asleep) short of the runway, and they will not reach their objective (a good night's sleep). They get only one chance in a glider and they'd better make it count!

As is generally true with behavioral approaches, compliance is an important issue with sleep restriction therapy. Therefore, while we have a clear conception of the general form of the treatment, we strive for a collaborative relationship in setting the particulars. After calculating what the initial schedule should be according to the sleep log, we ask patients if they can live with these bedtimes. Alterations to the schedule suggested by patients are made if they do not betray the spirit of the method. Patients are told that if they find that the schedule does not work for them, they should not change it on their own. Any alteration in the regimen must be discussed by the patient and the doctor so that hasty, ill-conceived decisions are avoided.

Between visits, patients telephone an answering machine in the morning to report the following:

1. The time they got into bed
2. How long it took to fall asleep
3. When they finally got out of bed in the morning
4. An estimate of how much they slept
5. Napping and alcohol intake

These daily reports serve many functions, which include keeping the clinician on top of the patients' progress, permitting timely interventions such as increasing time in bed, and letting patients know that the clinician is continually involved in their care.

If a patient does not abide by the schedule agreed upon, it is best if he or she is called on that day. Sometimes patients just need encouragement to make the extra effort, drag themselves out of bed in the morning, and put up with the daytime problems that occur in the first few weeks of treatment. When the schedule is repeatedly not followed, we explore what factors are contributing to the resistance. In addition to specific interpretations and interventions that indicate our understanding, we attempt to motivate patients in this situation by telling them that not everyone is able to comply with the standard treatment. In those cases, the treatment must be modified or combined with other interventions.

CASE 1: MRS. L

The first contact over the phone with Mrs. L was hampered by the patient's hearing problem combined with the malfunction of her telephone amplification system. I assumed she was fragile and that the hearing problem would interfere with therapy, given that the telephone is an important means of contact throughout the treatment. With misgivings, I scheduled an interview.

In marked contrast to my initial impression, Mrs. L presented as a very attractive, vigorous, well-spoken, self-assured woman. Humbled by the revelation of my ageism, I nonetheless pressed on. Mrs. L, an 80-year-old white, married, retired schoolteacher, complained of "difficulty falling asleep . . . [and] frequent awakening" which began four and a half years earlier, when her husband's Alzheimer's disease was diagnosed, and worsened four months before our interview, when he was placed in a nursing home. She was referred by a support group for spouses of Alzheimer's patients.

Mrs. L's medication regimen was as follows: thyroid, two grains per day, as replacement postthyroidectomy 50 years ago; Nicobid, dosage unreported, twice a day for the past 15 years, for "falling"; Timoptic and Pilocar for glaucoma; Proloid, one gram three times a day, for "metabolism"; and Lysine, for the past two years, for herpes.

A two-week sleep log indicated a severe insomnia (see Figures 1 and 2). Sleep latencies of two and a half hours, wakefulness of about three hours after sleep onset, and total sleep times of four hours were estimated. Mrs. L felt she spent more time awake in bed than asleep (sleep efficiencies of approximately 40 percent). The log indicated average time in bed to be slightly less than ten hours. Mrs. L did not complain of significant daytime drowsiness.

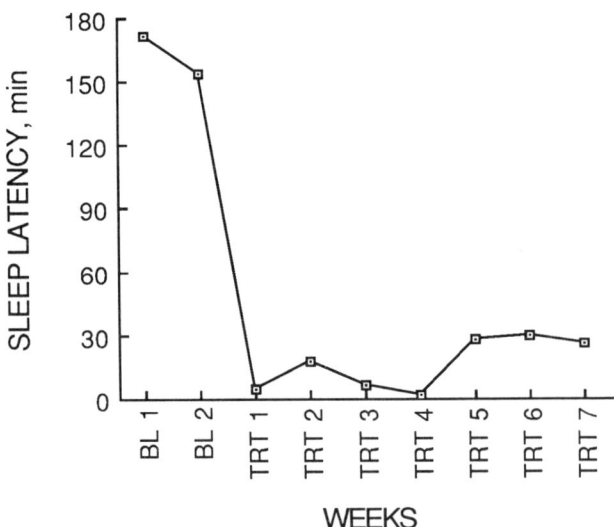

Figure 1. Mrs. L's mean weekly sleep latency, as reported on a sleep log during the two-week baseline (BL) and seven weeks of treatment (TRT).

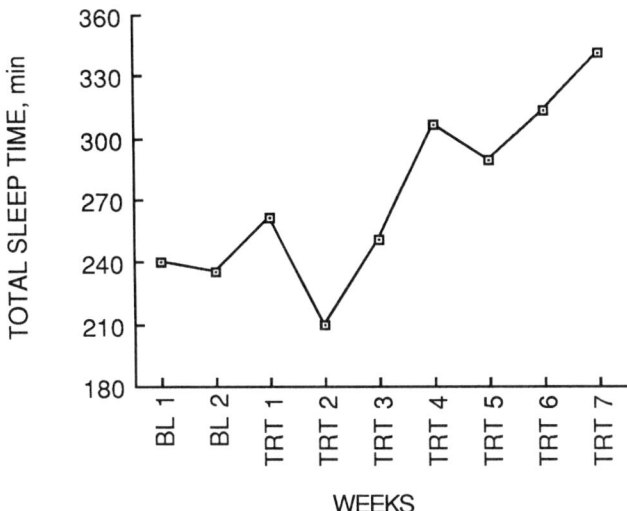

Figure 2. Mrs. L's mean weekly total sleep time, as reported on a sleep log during the two-week baseline (BL) and seven weeks of treatment (TRT).

On the four consecutive nights that Mrs. L spent in a sleep laboratory, her complaints and sleep log reports were only partly borne out (Table 1). Sleep latency to stage 2 was long at 41 minutes, and wakefulness during the sleep period was high at 71 minutes. Stage 4 was virtually absent, and sleep in general was severely fragmented (Figure 3). Sleep time was not short as subjectively reported; in fact, it totaled nearly eight hours! We presume that the numerous interruptions of sleep and predominantly lighter stages of sleep contributed to the perception of little sleep. Multiple sleep latency testing confirmed her subjective report of daytime alertness, with a mean sleep latency of 13.1 minutes (Table 2).

Mrs. L was prescribed an initial time in bed of 4.5 hours. In the first week of treatment, subjective parameters of sleep latency, wakefulness after sleep onset, and sleep efficiency (sleep duration/time in bed × 100 percent) all improved dramatically. These improvements were maintained over the course of the seven-week treatment, as time in bed was gradually increased to seven hours. Overall, Mrs. L estimated that her sleep time increased from 4 to 5.5 hours.

Mrs. L reported frequent drowsiness and occasional napping during the first week of treatment. This daytime sleepiness intensified during the second week of treatment. A Multiple Sleep Latency Test conducted after one week of treatment yielded an average sleep latency of 2.6 minutes,

Table 1. Nocturnal Sleep Recording, Mrs. L[a]

	Pretreatment (mean of nights 2 and 3)		End of treatment (mean of nights 2 and 3)	
Time in bed	581		421	
Sleep Latency (Stage 2)	41		2	
Wake after sleep onset	71		26	
Stage 1, min, % of TST	42	9.0	31	7.8
Stage 2, min, % of TST	331	70.4	234	59.4
Stage 3, min, % of TST	20	4.3	29	7.4
Stage 4, min, % of TST	0	0	21	5.4
Stage REM, Min, % of TST	77	16.3	79	20.0
Total sleep time	470		393	
Sleep efficiency	80.9		93.3	

[a]TST = total sleep time; TIB = time in bed; Sleep efficiency = TST/TIB × 100 percent

reflecting extreme daytime sleepiness. Trooper that she was, Mrs. L hardly needed encouragement to continue. Her weekly questionnaires indicated benefits from treatment almost immediately. She no longer awoke at night, worried and anxious; she no longer dwelled on what her night's sleep would bring; and she no longer reported restless sleep interrupted by long awakenings. After three weeks of treatment, Mrs. L's Multiple Sleep Latency Test levels had improved somewhat, to a still sleepy 4.8 minutes.

Nocturnal polysomnography conducted after six weeks showed a greatly improved sleep latency of two minutes and reduced wakefulness after sleep onset of 26 minutes (Figure 4). Stage 4 sleep, virtually absent at

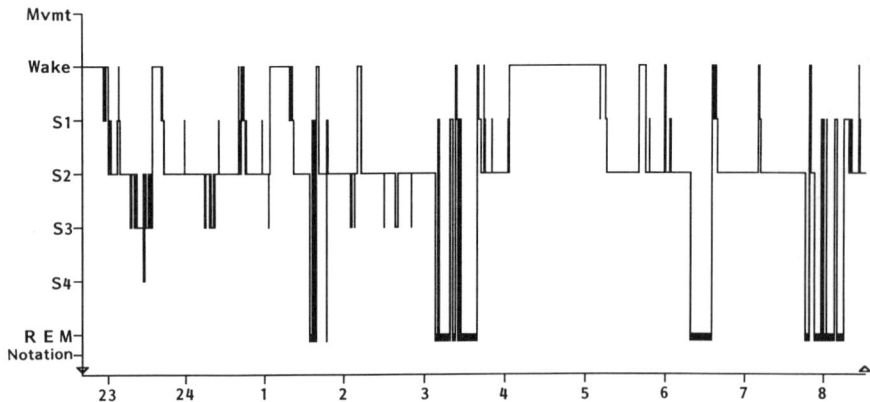

Figure 3. Mrs. L prior to sleep restriction therapy, spending an inordinate amount of time in bed. Sleep is fragmented with brief and long periods of wakefulness.

Table 2. Multiple Sleep Latency[a] Test, Mrs. L

	Pretreatment	Week 1	Week 3	End of treatment
Mean sleep latency (min)	13.1	2.6	4.8	5.2
Number of sleep latency < 5 min	1	5	3	2

[a]Sleep latency is defined as the duration from lights out to the first occurrence of three consecutive episodes of stage 1 or one epoch of any other stage of sleep.

baseline, was present for an average of 21 minutes over two nights. Sleep efficiency increased to 93 percent. However, total sleep time was reduced by 77 minutes, and daytime sleepiness, as assessed by the Multiple Sleep Latency Test, was still significant at 5.2 minutes.

While Mrs. L was unequivocal in her enthusiasm regarding the treatment outcome, at the point at which the protocol dictated that sleep recordings be performed, she was still improving. Both her reported and objective sleep efficiencies were over 90 percent, but she still required increased time in bed.

The treatment was, in fact, continued for three additional weeks. In reviewing questionnaires completed during this time, we found that the increased time in bed prescribed had ultimately led to increased sleep time of seven hours. Mrs. L's subjective drowsiness and incidence of napping were reduced. On the very last questionnaire, she reported, for the first time, "always" getting an adequate amount of sleep. Thus, while the early

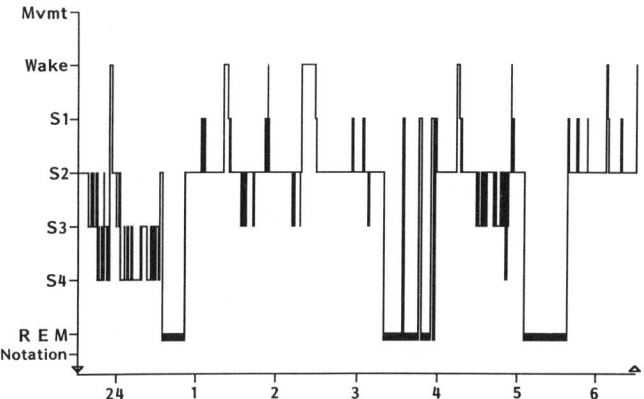

Figure 4. Mrs. L after six weeks of sleep restriction therapy. Her sleep period is compact and sleep is consolidated with the appearance of substantial slow-wave sleep.

phases of the treatment produced sleepiness, it is possible that a later recording would have been in accord with her reported increased nocturnal sleep time and reduced daytime sleepiness.

CASE 2: DIANE

Diane, a diminutive young woman wearing a stylish dress, arrived just in time for the initial consultation. Even so, she apologized for her tardiness. When informed that she was not a minute late, she responded, "Oh, I thought that before the first session you would want me to fill out a lot of papers." We began without filling out forms; Diane was seated on the edge of the couch, her chin resting on her hands, waiting for me to begin. She was experienced at first interviews, having worked as a personnel administrator in Massachusetts for several years before opting for graduate work in special education.

The presenting problem was insomnia. On good nights, it would take Diane what seemed to be an hour to fall asleep, and even then she would soon wake up and stay in bed fitfully, aware of the clock until early morning. She would get her "best sleep" between 5 and 7 A.M., but stay in bed until about 8:30 A.M. On other nights, there would be no sleep at all. She would get into bed around 11 P.M., and while lying there alone she would worry, either about minutia or about the general course of her life. Her advisor at school was inaccessible, her student loan was held up for some reason and her carburetor was out of adjustment. If she were going to finish her degree requirements in 1991, she would have to secure an externship soon. She had had a stupid argument with her boyfriend, Carl, over some theater tickets; she thought that he could afford to pay for them both on his salary. With these thoughts revolving around in her head, she would finally exhaust herself, reaching a halfway state between sleep and anxiety, and wait out the night.

Diane traced the onset of these sleep difficulties back three years, when a bout of pneumonia had gone undetected, followed by a serum reaction to an inoculation. The insomnia was accompanied by daytime lethargy and susceptibility to colds. Her coping capacities were exhausted when an AIDS test was recommended. (After her divorce, Diane had become involved with a man who later divulged a history of IV drug abuse.) It was two weeks before Diane received a negative result.

Oddly, when a specialist in Boston finally diagnosed a relatively mild case of congenital thyroid disorder and instituted appropriate treatment, Diane's relief was mixed with a continuing malaise. The several years devoted to medical consultations, the brush with the prospect of an early death, the decision to reorient her career toward learning disabilities and pursue a doctorate, all combined to make Diane feel that she had slipped backward or, at least, was not as far along on her career path as her family and friends in Northhampton would have predicted. Diane had been considered most likely to succeed all through high school, a brunette version of the golden girl who was going to demonstrate that career achievement and a marriage that worked were not mutually exclusive. Now the career was proving elusive, and the marriage was over. From this vantage point, 34 years of age seemed old to start catching up.

Diane was given a sleep log to fill out until the next session, listing the "Date," "Time In and Out of Bed," and "Hours Slept" to the nearest quarter-hour. This log showed her typical bedtime to be generally around midnight, somewhat later than what had first been reported. On Sunday night, bedtime had been delayed until 2:30 A.M. Typical rising times were 8:30 to 9:00 A.M. On three of the nights, Diane reported no sleep whatsoever. Other nights, she estimated her total sleep time to average around three hours.

Although Diane did not feel that her sleep added up to more than three or four hours at best, it was proposed that her typical nine-hour bedtime be shortened initially to six and a half hours. Seven and a half hours were allowed on the weekends as a "reward" for getting through the week. An even more rigorous schedule had been discussed, but Diane felt that she would have little success in complying with it and, in fact, doubted that she had the necessary discipline to follow the more lenient one.

The last hour of the evening before bedtime was designated a "buffer" period. During this time she could practice her relaxation exercises, listen to tranquil music, read, write letters, or watch television (apart from the 11 P.M. news or other anxiety-provoking features). She could not take calls from friends, including Carl. She could not do schoolwork, pay bills, or get involved in other activities that were likely to trigger an obsessive cycle.

While under treatment, Diane agreed to refrain from consuming any caffeinated beverage or sleeping medication. She was also advised to stop reading and watching television in bed. It was suggested that she arrange a divider in her studio apartment in order to better differentiate an area set aside for sleep.

The result of all these interventions was moderately encouraging. Diane was able to shorten her typical bedtime to seven hours. Even when she "cheated," she was out of bed by 8 A.M. Over the next two weeks, her average subjective sleep time was between three and four hours. Although this was a bit longer than before, she still felt that the sleep was "light." After having two arguments with Carl, she reported no sleep whatsoever.

Now that Diane could see for herself that a seven-hour bedtime was feasible, she was more amenable to slight additional reductions in bedtime. The need for these reductions was suggested by the continuing presence of several hours of subjective wakefulness during the night. Her bedtime was pushed back in two 15-minute increments to 12:30 A.M. Over the next few months, her subjective sleep time gradually increased to over four hours. The range of her subjective sleep time was between two and six hours. In other words, there were better nights, but there were also still very poor nights. Diane's sleep latency did not improve, she could spend one to two hours before falling asleep. However, she would then generally sleep through the night until the morning.

During the fourth month of treatment, Diane began to report bedtimes gradually increasing to seven hours or more, and she would appear at sessions (which were spaced two weeks apart) both apologetic and disappointed. She felt that her inability to maintain the schedule was further evidence of her ineffectiveness. She compensated for this lack of performance with meticulous and comprehensive record keeping, detailing not only her oversleeping, which she confessed as though it were a crime, but also food and beverage consumption, exercise periods, school assignments, alertness ratings, phases of her menstrual cycle, and arguments with Carl.

There was a clear enough correspondence between some of these factors and particular nights of poor sleep to suggest that a plateau had been reached. When life events were relatively calm, she could sleep five to six hours. Under the stress of a deadline or social tensions, cognitive intrusions would lower the subjective report to two hours. It was agreed that since the sleep restriction program was providing more opportunities for reproach than for efficient sleep, it would be discontinued in favor of a more relaxed recommendation of a seven-hour bedtime. Diane was nonetheless hesitant to relinquish her focus on each night's sleep length.

DISCUSSION

The case of Diane illustrates the potential conflicts between a narrow focus on a bedtime regimen and larger clinical issues, particularly with obsessive, perfectionistic characters. Sleep restriction therapy provided Diane with a convenient standard against which she could fall short. She could never adhere to it perfectly, and even when her compliance was acceptable, the treatment was not sufficiently effective, underscoring the special hopelessness of her situation.

Why didn't the treatment work? Its failure might be interpreted as evidence of the power of cognitive intrusions, which would call into question the decision to begin with only a moderately restricted schedule. In the initial stages of treatment, sleepiness can be a therapeutic ally against such intrusions; in Diane's case sleepiness was never allowed to accumulate full force. A second explanation for the treatment failure is that sleep restriction therapy, with its emphasis on self-monitoring, allowed free range to Diane's punctiliousness and tendency toward self-recrimination rather than holding a mirror to these character traits, traits that were also causing difficulties outside of treatment.

The cases presented in this chapter illustrate that sleep restriction therapy is not to be considered a mechanical procedure that can be administered with a telephone and a calculator. We are asking our patients to make drastic changes in their daily routines and to suffer through the pronounced side effects associated with sleep loss. Regular visits, timely phone calls, and flexibility informed by clinical judgment are all necessary for good results.

In particular, the clinician practicing sleep restriction therapy should not feel beholden to a mathematical formula. If an extra 15 minutes of bedtime is indicated more for motivation than because of sleep consolidation, it still should be considered. If the patient is overwhelmed by sleep loss, a first effort might be directed toward securing a two-week "trial period" for the beneficial effects of sleep consolidation to make an appearance, or deferring sleep restriction therapy altogether in favor of less demanding sleep hygiene or stimulus control measures.

Ultimately, the patient undergoing sleep restriction therapy will have to cope with sleep loss, as mild sleep deprivation is one of the "active ingredients" at the start of treatment. This loss triggers compensatory processes that strengthen sleep propensity. This is reflected by rapid sleep onset, consolidated sleep, deep sleep, and daytime sleepiness. Another contribution of the therapy stems from the string of rapid sleep onsets it produces. The repeated pairing of short sleep latency and bedtime cues strengthens their association; patients learn to fall asleep rapidly in their bedrooms.

Sleep restriction therapy also reduces the intensity of patients' anticipatory anxiety, the concern over what the night will bring. The concern fulfills its prophecy and disrupts the night, leading to a vicious cycle. Sleep restriction therapy ameliorates patients' anxiety by reducing the variability in the sleep that fuels it. Patients no longer experience the occasional sleep of their dreams, that nine-hour "rest cure," but, by the same token, their heightened sleep propensities offer some assurance against disastrous nights of little or no sleep. Routinely accumulating first about five and then six or seven hours of sleep removes the issue from the center of concern.

At the end of treatment, patients appreciate the gains they have made, but many do not feel confident about the future; they may still consider themselves "insomniacs." Follow-up at increasing intervals provides a helpful support and prepares the patient for any recurrence of insomnia. Rather than fearing a flareup, patients are encouraged to view it as an opportunity for demonstrating their mastery over the problem.

Paul B. Glovinsky received his doctorate in Clinical Psychology from the City College of the City University of New York where he is currently an Adjunct Assistant Professor in the Experimental Cognition Doctoral Program. Dr. Glovinsky has investigated mechanisms of daytime sleepiness, narcolepsy, and clinical and theoretical issues of insomnia. An accredited clinical polysomnographer, he was Staff Psychologist at the Montefiore Medical Center's Sleep–Wake Disorders Center for several years and is currently Co-Director of the Insomnia Treatment Center in New York City.

Arthur J. Spielman is Professor of Psychology, Head of the Experimental Cognition Doctoral Program, and Director of the Sleep Disorders Center at the City College of the City University of New York. He is a clinical psychologist and an accredited clinical polysomnographer with experience in the research, evaluation, and treatment of sleep disorders, specializing in the behavioral treatment of insomnia. Dr. Spielman was previously Co-Director of the Sleep–Wake Disorders Center at Montefiore Medical Center and is currently Co-Director of the Insomnia Treatment Center in New York City.

RECOMMENDED READINGS

Spielman, A. J., Caruso, L. S., & Glovinsky, P. B. (1987). A behavioral perspective on insomnia treatment. In M. Ermin (Ed.), *Psychiatric Clinics of North America*, Philadelphia: W. B. Saunders, pp. 541–553.
    This review paper places sleep restriction therapy within the context of the entire range of behavioral treatments for insomnia.
Spielman, A. J., Saskin, P., & Thorpy, M. J. (1987). Treatment of chronic insomnia by restriction of time in bed. *Sleep*, *10*(1), 45–56.
    The initial publication regarding sleep restriction, this paper details the technique and presents the outcome of a clinical case series.

REFERENCES

Bootzin, R. R., & Nicassio, P. M. (1978). Behavioral treatments for insomnia. In M. Hersen, R. M. Eisler, & P. M. Miller (Eds.). *Progress in behavior modification* (Vol. 6). New York: Academic Press, pp. 1–45.

Edinger, J. D., Hoelscher, T. J., Webb, M. D., Marsh, G. R., Radtke, R. A., & Erwin, C. W. (1989). Polysomnographic assessment of DIMS: Empirical evaluation of its diagnostic value. *Sleep, 12*(4), 315–322.

Friedman, L., Bliwise, D. L., Yesave, J. A., & Salom, S. R. (1990). A preliminary study comparing sleep restriction and relaxation treatments for insomnia in older adults. *Journal of Gerontology: Psychological Sciences, 46*, 1–8.

Morin, C., Kowatch, R., & Wade, J. (1989). Behavioral management of sleep disturbances secondary to chronic pain. *Journal of Behavior Therapy and Experimental Psychiatry, 20*(4), 295–302.

Morin C., Kowatch, R., & O'Shanick, G. (1990). Sleep restriction for the in-patient treatment of insomnia. *Sleep, 13*(2), 182–186.

Rubinstein, M. L., Rothenberg, S. A., Maheswaran, S., Tsai, J. S., Zozula, R., & Spielman, A. J. (1990). Modified sleep restriction therapy in middle-aged and elderly chronic insomniacs. *Sleep Research, 19*, 276.

Spielman, A. J. (1986). Assessment of insomnia. *Clinical Psychology Reviews, 6*, 11–25.

Spielman, A. J., Caruso, L., & Glovinsky, P. B. (1987). A behavioral perspective on insomnia treatment. In M. Ermin (Ed.). *Psychiatric Clinics of North America*. Philadelphia: W. B. Saunders, pp. 541–553.

Spielman, A. J., Saskin, P., & Thorpy, M. J. (1987). Treatment of chronic insomnia by restriction of time in bed. *Sleep, 10*(1), 45–56.

Webb, W., & Agnew, H. (1965). Sleep: Effects of a restricted regime. *Science, 150*, 1745–1747.

Webb, W., & Agnew, H. (1974). The effects of a chronic limitation of sleep length. *Psychophysiology, 11*, 265–274.

CHAPTER FIVE

Sleep Hygiene, Relaxation Therapy, and Cognitive Interventions

PETER J. HAURI

Sleep hygiene, relaxation therapy, and some cognitive interventions make a good package that can often be administered conjointly. I typically use an individualized mix of them in my initial treatment sessions with chronic insomniacs.

SLEEP HYGIENE

Advising those with insomnia on what to do is probably an activity as old as mankind, and much nonsense has been perpetuated in this area. However, over the last 30 years, a fairly substantial body of research has been accumulated to scientifically support a set of rules on how to get better sleep. I first summarized this body of evidence in 1977 (Hauri, 1977) and, for lack of a better term, I called it "sleep hygiene." The name stuck, although I have never liked it.

Giving advice on sleep hygiene is more difficult than is typically appreciated. I often tell patients the anecdote of how a few years ago I advised many insomniacs to take a leisurely stroll around the neighborhood before going to bed. It helped many of them. But then I encountered a businessman for whom that advice was quite detrimental. He slept very little during the week that he tried to follow it. He found that when he was

---

Peter J. Hauri • Sleep Disorders Center, Mayo Clinic, Rochester, Minnesota 55905.

strolling leisurely around his neighborhood, he started remembering all the forgotten details of his business day and started to ruminate about the missed opportunities of the day. By the time he returned home he was "wound tighter than a drum." Through trial and error, we found that this man slept best if, in the evening, he went to his basement, where he had a metal lathe and worked on tolerances of 1000th of a millimeter. After two hours of very exacting work in his metal hobby shop (work that would drive many others to nervous exhaustion), he felt relaxed and fell asleep easily. The point of the anecdote is that one person's "sleep elixir" may well be another person's poison. The task of matching sleep hygiene advice to the individual patient requires considerable clinical skill.

Many mental health professionals hand their patients little pamphlets filled with "sleep hygiene rules." This is no more effective, in my experience, than handing a neurotic patient a list of ten "rules for healthy emotional living." Rather, it is important for the therapist to keep these sleep hygiene rules in his or her own mind and use them judiciously when discussing the particular sleep problem with a patient. I have rarely found a patient who can benefit from more than three or four individually tailored rules at any given time.

Following are some sleep hygiene rules in a rough order of overall frequency with which I use them during my insomnia interviews:

1. *Curtail time in bed*: Assume that a person needs only six hours of sleep per night but stays in bed for eight. The result is usually not only a guaranteed two hours of sleeplessness, but, much more disturbing, over time there develops a generally more shallow sleep with many awakenings. Stage I sleep increases. In the morning such a person feels less restored than if he or she had slept for a solid six hours. The natural tendency then is to stay in bed even longer because one is still fatigued, which leads to even less restorative sleep, in a vicious cycle.

The almost universal need of insomniacs to curtail their bedtime forms the basis of sleep restriction therapy, discussed in this book by Drs. Glovinsky and Spielman. I use a much less drastic version in most of my cases. To assess a person's overall need to sleep, I make use of the facts that, in normal sleepers, overall sleep needs (over a 24-hour period) do not change much from age 20 to age 75 (Williams, Karacan, & Hursch, 1974). Thus, I first ask my patients how much they slept long before insomnia hit. (If they do not know, I ask whether as children they were exceptionally short or long sleepers. If they do not remember, I feel they probably were sleeping average lengths and, as adults, probably need about seven and a half hours.) I then recommend that bedtime be held solidly to that amount of time.

2. *Never try to sleep*: The more a person tries to sleep, the more aroused he or she gets. This was recognized by the ancients who recommended that insomniacs try counting sheep. They knew from experience with their own flocks that this was a very boring task which, nevertheless, absorbed attention and, therefore, kept the insomniac patients from trying too hard to sleep.

Because counting sheep is foreign to our culture, I typically replace it by prescribing either reading in bed, watching television, or listening to all-night talk shows. Patients are asked to do these activities in bed as long as they can possibly hold out. Paradoxically, the harder they try to stay awake, the easier it is to fall asleep. I am interested in developing a learned association between a bedroom behavior and sleep onset. If reading always leads to sleep, then, over a number of trials, sleeping becomes the conditioned response to reading in bed. However, it takes a few weeks to set up that response, and patients must read every night until they fall asleep, even if it takes them most of the night. Obviously, they still have to get up at their usual arousal times in the morning no matter how long they have read, and no naps are allowed during the day.

In two other chapters in this book, Bootzin, Epstein, and Wood, as well as Lacks, discuss stimulus control therapy, a successful technique of sleep induction that forbids patients to read or watch television in bed. I have found both their techniques and mine to work, although, I feel, with somewhat differential effectiveness, depending on the patient. Patients who have difficulties falling asleep when they try to do so, but fall asleep easily when they try to stay awake (e.g., in lectures, while driving, watching television, reading), seem to benefit more from my technique of reading or watching television in bed because that keeps them from trying too hard to sleep. Patients who show conditioned arousal to the bedroom, i.e., those who sleep best away from their own bedrooms, appear to benefit more from stimulus control therapy.

3. *Eliminate the bedroom clock*: It seems impossible to relax in bed when one knows that it is 3 A.M., that the minutes are ticking away, and that one will have to get up at 6 A.M. for a hard day's work. Yet, most insomniacs have illuminated bedroom clocks which they consult anxiously throughout the night. Time pressures are not conducive to sleep, and I have my patients set their alarm clocks and then put them underneath the bed, in the top dresser drawer, or somewhere else where they can neither see them nor hear them ticking. From then on, until the alarm rings, it is irrelevant what time it is. It is simply time to relax and/or sleep, no matter what the clock would say. A time-free environment seems helpful to falling asleep and staying asleep.

4. *Exercise in the late afternoon or early evening*: Sleep is tied to the

circadian rhythm, which is measured most easily by assessing core temperature. We seem to sleep best during the trough in our temperature curve. However, insomniacs seem to have a flatter circadian rhythm (less difference between peak and trough) than good sleepers (Lack, Kalucy, & Balfour, 1988). Intense exercise leads to an increase in core body temperature and to a compensatory drop in this temperature four to six hours later (Horne & Staff, 1983). This is the reason why morning exercise has no effect on sleep; the compensatory drop in temperature occurs during the afternoon and dissipitates by evening. However, intense exercise in the late afternoon or early evening, at least 20 minutes in the aerobic "target zone" (a heart rate increase adjusted for the age of the exerciser), leads to a rebound cooling around midnight and to better sleep.

Horne and Reid (1985) have shown that a similar effect can be achieved by passive heating, i.e., by staying in hot baths for at least 30 minutes. However, it appears that the compensatory drop in core temperature comes somewhat earlier after passive heating, i.e., about two to four hours later. Thus, if the patient cannot exercise around dinnertime, he or she might catch up by taking a hot bath two to four hours before going to bed.

5. *Avoid coffee, alcohol, and nicotine*: Coffee clearly disturbs sleep, even in those patients who do not experience such an effect (Karacan, Thornby, Anch, *et al.*, 1976). There is some evidence that insomniacs are often much more sensitive to caffeine or other mild stimulants (tea, chocolate) than are normal sleepers. Therefore, patients who have problems with sleeping should avoid coffee, caffeine-containing sodas, tea, or occasionally even chocolate, at least for the period between lunch and sleep. The same goes for smoking because tobacco, too, is a mild stimulant.

Low doses of alcohol do promote sleep onset (Rundell, Lester, Griffiths, *et al.*, 1972). Unfortunately, as the alcohol is metabolized, sleep becomes more fragmented and disturbed (Adamson & Burdick, 1973). This is why alcohol is not recommended as a hyponotic.

6. *Regularized bedtime*: Our internal circadian rhythm is not exactly 24 hours long. There is considerable evidence that in younger years (adolescence through early adulthood), the innate circadian rhythm is much longer than 24 hours. In old age, on the other hand, it occasionally becomes shorter than 24 hours (Czeisler, Rios, Sanchez, Brown, Richardson, Ronda, & Rogacz, 1986). In other words, for the young adult, when the clock on the wall indicates that it is midnight, his or her own body clock might indicate that it is only 9 P.M., and going to sleep would then be difficult. For the elderly, when the clock on the wall says that it is only 9 P.M., the internal body clock, being fast, might indicate midnight, and such a person would be very sleepy. This is why younger patients often

have difficulty falling asleep and getting up in the morning, while many elderly patients go to bed very early and then are unable to sleep after 3 or 4 A.M.

Because the innate circadian rhythm in the younger patients is usually longer than 24 hours and needs to be squeezed into a shorter time period every day, young adults need to keep a regular arousal time slightly before they are totally slept out. There is no use telling them to go to bed at a certain time. Rather, bedtime will gradually regulate itself if they rise at the regular time. On the other time, because the elderly often have to stretch a foreshortened circadian rhythm into the required 24 hours, they have to go to bed regularly and at a time that is later than comfortable. Wakeup time will then regulate itself, if the problem is truly circadian.

7. *Eat a light bedtime snack*: From numerous experiments in both animals and humans, we know that hunger can disrupt sleep (Jacobs & McGinty, 1971; Crisp & Stonehill, 1973). A light bedtime snack, such as a glass of warm milk or cheese and crackers, is clearly helpful (Southwell, Evans, & Hunt, 1972). The mechanism for this effect is disputed. Some claim that digestive hormones have a sedative effect (Fara, Rubinstein, & Sonnenschein, 1969), but others feel that the tryptophan in the bedtime snack might be involved.

8. *Explore napping*: Clinically, there are clearly different types of nappers. For some, a nap in the afternoon disturbs sleep that night. Others, however, sleep much better if they have allowed themselves an afternoon nap, possibly because after such a nap they do not need to sleep so much and, therefore, do not seek it so desperately. I advise all my patients to experiment with naps if this is possible in their daily schedule. They each take a nap each day for one week and keep track of their nighttime sleep. They then each eliminate the nap for a week and do the same. Averaging the total hours slept each night, the sleep latency, the number of awakenings, and so forth should tell them whether or not, in their case, they should try to nap.

9. *Hypnotics*: In Chapter Eight of this book, Stepanski *et al.* argue that hypnotics should either be given regularly for an entire month, or not at all. By doing this they try to avoid frequent rebound effects (when patients sleep more poorly than usual because they are withdrawing from hypnotics), and they try to eliminate the patients' nightly struggle over whether or not they should take pills. There is much clinical wisdom in that recommendation. Nevertheless, I have found that, in occasional patients, a rare prn (*pro re nata*) hypnotic as needed seems indicated. After discussing rebound insomnia [even after one night on Halcion (Merlotti, Roehrs, Zorick, Stepanski, Russo, & Roth, 1988)] with such patients, I recommend that they keep a few hypnotics and use them either after they have had

three consecutive very poor nights or on the night before a very important event (e.g., giving a talk, getting married, etc.). In either case, they need to take the hypnotic upon retiring, not in the middle of the night. In this way I try to avoid getting patients into the vicious cycle of sleeping poorly for a few nights, then needing sleep more and more desperately, and, therefore, keeping themselves from sleeping.

RELAXATION THERAPY

Numerous relaxation techniques have been shown to be more effective than credible placebo when treating sleep-onset insomnia. These techniques include progressive relaxation, i.e., a method of tensing and relaxing various muscle groups throughout the body (Coursey, Frankel, Gaarder, and Mott, 1980; Nicassio, Boylan, & McCabe, 1982); autogenic training, i.e., a complex technique of focusing one's attention on various parts of the body, coupled with self-suggestions of heaviness, warmth, etc.; meditation (Woolfolk, Carr-Kaffashan, McNulty, and Lehrer, 1976); abdominal breathing; and biofeedback (Hauri, 1981).

However, it may not be the actual amount of muscle relaxation that is crucial. Based on a series of well-controlled studies, Borkovec and Fowles (1973) concluded that learning to focus one's attention on relatively pleasant, monotonous, internal sensations may be incompatible with worrisome thoughts and images that prevent sleep onset. This cognitive refocusing may be the sleep-inducing mechanism rather than the actual tension that is released, according to Borkovec.

I have shown (Hauri, 1981) that not all insomniacs are psychologically or physiologically tense. Those who are relaxed but are still unable to sleep may actually become worse when pushed into relaxation training (Hauri, Percy, Hellekson, Hartmann, & Russ, 1982). Thus, it seems crucial to first assess how tense a person is before prescribing relaxation training.

There are different kinds of tension (e.g., psychological tension, muscle tension, sympathetic arousal, etc.), and they do not correlate more than about 0.40 with each other. Thus, it is quite possible that a person is muscularly tense while psychologically relaxed.

It would be ideal to assess the different forms of tensions right before sleep onset because there are some patients who may be relaxed all day only to become tense when faced with the task of going to sleep. Because this is very cumbersome, I have found it advantageous to assess at least frontalis muscle tension and hand temperature during the intake interview. I use standard biofeedback equipment, but without any biofeedback tone. A patient is first asked to simply lie down without being given any directions. Five minutes later he or she is asked to "relax as deeply as possible, just as if you wanted to sleep." Not only is the average level of frontalis electromyogram (EMG) or hand temperature of interest, but its change with time is as well. Is the patient relaxed when no demands are made, but tenses considerably as soon as relaxation is demanded? Does the patient relax deeper and deeper over a course of five minutes, or does the patient become more and more tense as time progresses?

If high muscle tension or a decreasing hand temperature is found, I typically start with a course in abdominal breathing because this method usually leads to results in one or two sessions. If it is not successful, I switch to progressive relaxation or biofeedback. These methods are practiced at home by the patients for at least one-half hour each day. Initially, I forbid them to use relaxation techniques at sleep onset, so as not to associate these techniques with failure. Only when the skills have developed and deep relaxation can be achieved on demand are the patients allowed to use these techniques when trying to fall asleep, or during the night when they have awakened.

COGNITIVE STRATEGIES

There is no question that maladaptive cognitions are at the root of many insomnias. It is hard to sleep when one fears the night, expecting that one will not sleep at all, or when one focuses on sleep with all one's might, trying to will oneself to sleep.

Techniques to combat maladaptive cognitions have been described in detail by Beck (1970) and by Ellis (1975). Many of them can be transferred directly to the treatment of insomnia.

An important principle in many cognitive therapies is to enlist the patient as "coscientist" (Meichenbaum, 1977). Instead of passively listening to the advice of the experts, I ask patients to make and test their own recommendations. A sleep log and a day log are important tools in this procedure (see Figures 1 and 2). In the sleep log, the patients note every morning how they slept. In the day log, patients keep track of four activities which, in their opinion, might be related to sleep quality. For example, if the patient feels that sleep is directly influenced by stress at work, this stress is noted and rated on a scale from 0 to 10 every night *before* the patient goes to sleep. After the patient has kept day logs and night logs for a week or two, one can evaluate whether or not there is actually a relationship.

I am at my therapeutic best if I can enlist the patient to recommend what should be logged. The patient knows best what might possibly affect

Sleep Log

Please fill out this Sleep Log every morning about 30 minutes after getting up. Guess the approximate times. Do not worry if your figures are not absolutely correct. We are interested in your opinion of how you slept. Date the night when it started, not when you fill it out (for example, if you filled the log out on Wednesday morning, Oct. 5, the date of the night is Tuesday, Oct. 4).

Name _____

DATE	SUN.	MON.	TUES.	WED.	THURS.	FRI.	SAT.
Did you take naps yesterday? If yes, give total length of sleep in minutes.							
Did you take any sleeping medication? Give time and amount.							
When did you turn out your lights, actually trying to sleep?							
How many minutes did it take you to fall asleep last night?							
How often did you awaken last night?							
How many minutes were you awake during last night? Do not count the time it took you to fall asleep initially.							
When did you wake up for the last time this morning?							
How many hours did you actually sleep last night?							
When did you get out of bed for the last time this morning?							
Compared with your own avg. over the last month, how well did you sleep last night? Choose one from the list below, left.							
Overall, how refreshing and restorative was your sleep? Choose one from the list below, right.							

1. Much worse than my average
2. Slightly worse than my average
3. Fairly typical for me
4. Slightly better than my average
5. Much better than my average

1. Not at all restorative—derived no benefit from my time in bed
2. Some slight restorative value
3. Restorative, but not adequately so
4. Relatively satisfactory
5. Very satisfactory—feel completely refreshed and ready for the day

Figure 1. Sleep log. (Reprinted by permission from Hauri & Linde, 1990.)

DAY LOG

Name _____

Date				
Sunday				
Monday				
Tuesday				
Wednesday				
Thursday				
Friday				
Saturday				

Figure 2. Day log. (Reprinted by permission from Hauri & Linde, 1990.)

sleep. I am often surprised what phenomena are finally discovered to affect the patient's sleep. With one patient it was a nightly telephone call from mother that affected sleep latency and that had to be changed to a morning telephone call. Another patient found that a calcium tablet taken around suppertime facilitated sleep. (I have no idea why such a tablet might be effective, and I do not generally recommend it.) Or it might be arguments that are carried out around bedtime that need to be changed to another time, or the habit of drinking a beer or two in the evening, etc. Even more important than finding such relationships and then changing the behavior is the new attitude of the patient. Instead of being a helpless victim of insomnia who has to be cured by the doctor, the patient now becomes an active collaborator in the task of finding solutions to a circumscribed problem.

CASE HISTORY (SUCCESSFUL)

Mrs. O was a 45-year-old homemaker and a wife of a high-school teacher. The couple had three children. Mr. and Mrs. O were highly respected in the community because both did much volunteer work and were always willing to contribute either time or money to worthwhile causes.

When I saw Mrs. O, she seemed exhausted. She had no idea why she could not sleep. Asked how she had spent last evening and night, she related that she had worked up to about 10 P.M. for various volunteer causes. The couple had gone to bed at 10:15 P.M., although she was not tired at that time. It then took her over one hour to fall asleep, partly because of her husband's loud snoring, partly because of her "jerkitis." By this she meant that often, when she tried to fall asleep, she experienced uncomfortable feelings in her calves, knees, and thighs which disappeared only with vigorous knee bending. More rarely, when she tried to relax, her legs repeatedly twitched involuntarily.

Last night Mrs. O fell asleep shortly before midnight and then awakened around 1:30 A.M. and around 4 A.M. Each awakening was followed by at least 45 minutes of wakefulness. During this time Mrs. O had stayed in bed planning her days, worrying about unfinished business, but mainly trying desperately to sleep. She related how she felt like a personal failure because of this insomnia.

Mrs. O felt that she got less than five hours of sleep before she finally arose at 6:30 A.M. this morning, tired and exhausted. She also felt that last night had been typical for her. She rarely took naps during the day but found that "a few cups" of coffee helped her get through the day. Occasionally, she did doze off in meetings, and she dreaded going to movies because she rarely saw more than the first half-hour before she fell asleep.

According to Mrs. O, she had "always" been a poor sleeper. As a child, she remembered many a night when she listened to her parents' conversations because she was not sleepy but was forbidden to read in bed. As far as she remembered, no specific traumas were associated with her childhood insomnia. Insomnia had gradually grown worse over her adult life and had become quite serious during the last five years.

Mrs. O did little exercise, mainly because she felt too busy. She drank alcohol only rarely. Asked to keep track of her coffee intake for a week, she reported an average of seven cups of coffee per day, almost evenly spaced throughout the day. Asked what she has tried so far to help her improve her sleep, she reported that for a number of years she had tried desperately each night to think only pleasant thoughts, but that unhappy thoughts had always intruded when she was almost falling asleep. This, too, contributed to her feeling that she was weak-willed or "bad."

As part of the insomnia assessment, a psychophysiological evaluation of frontalis EMG and finger temperature was carried out. Mrs. O first was asked to lie down and move very little, "while we are calibrating the equipment." During this time, her frontalis EMG was medium-high, and her hand temperature remained steady at 82.4°F. She was then asked to relax as deeply as she could. Over the next five minutes, her frontalis EMG gradually rose to very high levels, while her hand temperature decreased by 0.6°F.

Because of the possibility that insomnia was associated with periodic leg movements and the restless-legs syndrome, Mrs. O was studied in the laboratory for one night. During that night she fell asleep in 15 minutes and slept a total of six and one-half hours. She was aware and embarrassed that she had slept much better in the lab than at home. There were frequent periodic leg movements during the first two hours of the night, and many aroused Mrs. O.

Summarizing all the findings, I felt that Mrs. O's insomnia was complex. There certainly was a predisposition toward poor sleep, as indicated by her sleep problems in childhood. There was a learned component, suggested by her sleeping so much better in the lab than at home. There was an inability to relax, documented by her frontalis EMG and hand temperature during the psychophysiological assessment. There was excessive caffeine intake. Restless legs and periodic leg movements aggravated the insomnia. Nevertheless, it seemed likely to me that excessive stress played the major role in this problem, and I had the distinct impression that there were some psychological issues that had not yet surfaced.

I decided to start treatment with a program of sleep hygiene and relaxation training. The hope was that such a program would give some early relief from Mrs. O's insomnia, making her more willing to consider psychological issues later on. A decision concerning medication, either for insomnia or for her restless-leg syndrome and periodic leg movements, was deferred to a later date.

In the first therapy session, we discussed the fact that different people have different needs for sleep and that she might not need the slightly more than eight hours of sleep that her husband required. We suggested that she go to bed only when sleepy and that she get up in the morning when she felt that she had slept enough.

To my surprise, this suggestion resulted in an angry phone call from her husband who could not understand what we were trying to do. He finally agreed that it did not help him if his wife lay in bed awake while he was asleep. The suggestion was then modified so that the couple would go to bed together but that Mrs. O was allowed to get up if she did not feel sleepy once he was soundly asleep. Because of Mrs. O's observation that she often fell asleep when trying to stay awake, we suggested that when unable to sleep, Mrs. O should go to another bedroom and read. She was told that, while sleeping was clearly best, reading while relaxing in bed was much more restorative than being tense and frustrated, tossing and turning.

Because of Mrs. O's constant thinking and planning when awake during the night, I suggested a procedure called "worry time." She was told that, in my judgment, she did not think or plan too much, but that she did it at the wrong time. She was asked to withdraw to a quiet room for about one-half hour each evening, at least two hours before bedtime. There she was to sit in a comfortable chair, holding a stack of 3×5 cards and letting her mind wander without really trying to worry. If there were untoward thoughts, things that needed to be planned, or concerns that needed to be addressed, she was to write each thought on one of the 3×5 cards. When no more such thoughts appeared, Mrs. O was asked to sort the cards into three to seven piles according to their content, e.g., all financial thoughts together, all thoughts concerning relationships, etc. (Such an ordering of the thoughts into content areas often brings some control into the chaos of innumerable worries swirling uncontrollably around one's head.) After that, each thought was to be contemplated with the goal of developing a solution. If a solution was found, it had to be written down on that particular card. For example, if tomorrow was going to be a particularly busy day, Mrs. O was to write out a plan for that day. If the concern was that she had $800 worth of bills but only $200 to pay them, she was to write down right then which bills were to be paid, which would receive only a down payment, and which would simply be deferred for next month. In cases where no solution could be found, Mrs. O was to write on the card, in longhand, a phrase like "I have thought about this problem carefully but cannot find a solution today." I have often found that thinking and worrying in this systematized way during the evening clears an obsessive worrier's head during awakenings from sleep.

Mrs. O was also informed about the beneficial effects of early-evening exercise, both on sleep and on some types of the restless-leg syndrome. After considerable discussion, she was enrolled in a fitness class at the local YWCA which met from 4:30 P.M. to 5:30 P.M.

Finally, Mrs. O was informed about the role of caffeine in the restless-leg syndrome, in periodic leg movements, and in insomnia. She agreed to a gradual tapering program, down to two cups in the morning.

During the intake, Mrs. O had been given a sleep log to write down when she went to bed, how long it took her to fall asleep, when she awakened, etc. She filled out this log to the minute. This indicated that she was an anxious clock watcher, and I asked her to eliminate the bedroom clock.

In the second session, Mrs. O reported some marginal progress. She was then introduced to abdominal breathing, a guided relaxation exercise. She seemed enthusiastic and was asked to rehearse this procedure daily for one-half hour. According to the log she brought to the third session, she did so for the first four days and then stopped rehearsing. Queried about this, she admitted that the relaxation training made her uncomfortable and unhappy. Once it had even triggered a flood of tears, for unknown reasons. Such negative reactions to relaxation are not rare. In Mrs. O's case, I simply interpreted these events as showing that Mrs. O was now able to enter a deeper state of relaxation where a number of unhappy, pent-up feelings could gradually be released. Mrs. O was supported to continue, and to let the unhappy feelings take their course.

Over a number of sessions, we worked with the day log/night log paradigm. Each session Mrs. O selected four possible factors that might influence her insomnia. She then rated those factors each evening of the next week on a scale from 0 to 10. She also filled out the sleep log each morning. During the following session we tried to assess whether a certain factor might have had any influence on sleep. With this procedure we found that arguments after 8 P.M. were quite detrimental to her sleep, as was work of any kind after about 9 P.M. However, it then took considerable work on my part to have Mrs. O realize that at least one hour per day, if not more, should be spent in leisure activities that were not immediately productive, but simply pleasant for her. Finally, having been an English major, she started to enjoy a number of books she had always wanted to read but had felt that there was no time for. However, this "wasted time" before bedtime made her feel guilty, especially since she experienced considerable pressure from her husband to use her time more productively.

During the fifth therapy session, my sleep hygiene advice clashed openly with her husband's opinion on how one's life should be lived. Therefore, he was invited for the next session. After I had defined the purpose of my work with his wife as trying to look into any area that might keep her from sleeping soundly, I invited each to listen to the other in an attempt to better understand each other's concerns. To my surprise, the husband started first by forcefully expressing his disgust for having a weak-willed wife who had recently started to become selfish when there was such a need for doing good in this world. Shocked, she immediately tried to make peace by offering to jettison her reading and by her returning to her previous eight-hour ordeal of insomnia in the marital bed. I objected that, initially, it was more important to understand each other rather than following a shortcut into action. Three hours of intense marital therapy followed before better communication was established and each partner felt somewhat freer to be him/herself.

At the end of my work, the question of medication for Mrs. O's restless-leg syndrome and periodic leg movements was raised again. Mrs. O declined any medication, feeling that her "jerkitis" had much improved. Although there is no research basis for it, I have frequently noticed that the type of periodic leg movements that occurs only at the beginning of the night is quite responsive to exercise and to decreasing caffeine, possibly because circulatory issues may be involved.

Throughout the eight sessions that I saw Mrs. O, she filled out sleep logs. They documented an initial marked increase in total sleep, a gradual further increase as the behavioral parts were put into place, a deterioration of sleep during the marriage therapy, but a gradual improvement thereafter. I then lost track of Mrs. O until I placed a follow-up telephone call to her one year later. Mrs. O said that sleep was still an occasional problem but that the problem was nowhere near the severity it had been when she sought my help.

I selected this case history for a number of reasons. First, it makes the point that insomnia is usually quite complex and multidetermined. Also, the goal of therapy may change; there was no evidence at the beginning that marital strife was underlying Mrs. O's insomnia, mainly because most of the community saw them as an ideal couple. Also, even if such psychological issues do underline insomnia, in those who deny problems, it is often better to start with behavioral therapy and sleep hygiene. After some initial progress, a patient starts to trust the therapist and may be more willing to engage in other explorations. This is particularly important because insomniacs are often repressors, denying emotional problems both to themselves and to others. Obviously there are many other cases where sleep hygiene and relaxation training are all that is needed, without further therapeutic work.

CASE HISTORY (UNSUCCESSFUL)

Miss B, a 26-year-old student at a local community college, was referred to the Sleep Disorders Center for a combination of insomnia and excessive daytime sleepiness.

Currently, Miss B went to bed around midnight and then needed two or three hours before she could fall asleep. Her sleep was quite fragmented and shallow, with many long awakenings until about 6 A.M. Her best sleep typically came from 6 to 8 A.M. when her alarm sounded. From then until 11 A.M., Miss B would lie in bed, dozing on and off but feeling too tired to get up. In anticipation of this, she had registered only for afternoon and evening courses, which she usually attended, although she occasionally dozed off in them. She typically took a nap around 6 P.M. and then seemed to become more and more alert as the evening progressed.

Miss B had been a lively teenager until she was about 14, when she was involved in a serious car accident and sustained multiple injuries. The most obvious chronic handicap stemming from that accident was a severely limping gait. There was also some kidney damage and some head trauma, leaving her with a mild memory deficit. Miss B also suffered chronic pain in a number of her joints.

At the time of the referral, Miss B lived alone in an apartment close to her parents, who were quite involved in her life. She had a live-in boyfriend, a student from the same community college. Miss B had an adequate income from the settlement of the accident. Although she claimed that her goal in life was to become a clinical psychologist, she had not managed to graduate from the two-year community college she had attended for the last four years. Her pattern was to start a number of courses with high enthusiasm but to drop most of them sometime before finals. Typically, the reason given for withdrawal was either excessive pain or insomnia.

At the time of our interview, Miss B drank two cups of coffee around noon and one to three beers in the evening "to relax." She did not engage in any exercise. The Minnesota Multiphasic Personality Inventory was within normal limits except for scales 1 and 3, which were elevated above 70, in part due to her numerous somatic complaints and disabilities.

As part of the insomnia assessment, a psychophysiological assessment of frontalis EMG and hand temperature was carried out. Initially, both were well within normal limits, until I asked Miss B to relax. After that, frontalis EMG increased quite markedly and steadily rose over the next five minutes. Hand temperature dropped by about 2°F during the same period.

Other aspects of Miss B's sleep history were well within normal limits, except that her boyfriend complained that she snored loudly. There were no signs of narcolepsy (e.g., cataplexy, hypnagogic hallucinations, or sleep paralysis), and there were no parasomnias, such as sleepwalking, nightmares, or bedwetting.

In the past, Miss B had been put on hypnotics (Halcion, 0.25 mg) during the night and on stimulants (Ritalin, 20 mg) during the day. According to her, these medications had had very little effect.

Because of Miss B's excessive daytime sleepiness, her snoring, and her chronic pain, which might be related to alpha/delta sleep, she was studied in the lab for one night. She went to bed around midnight, fell asleep around 2:30 A.M., and then slept intermittently until 10:30 A.M. There were numerous awakenings. There was no delta sleep (the deepest sleep of the night). Miss B was snoring moderately, but there were no disordered breathing events, and there were no periodic leg movements. There was no excessive alpha during non–rapid eye movement sleep. In summary, Miss B had about seven hours of normal, but shallow, sleep with frequent awakenings during ten hours of bedtime.

Because of her excessive daytime sleepiness, we also did a multiple sleep latency test. Miss B stayed in the lab for the day after her sleep evaluation and was asked to take a nap four times, at two-hour intervals. In her case, the naps were scheduled at noon, 2 P.M., 4 P.M., and 6 P.M. Miss B fell asleep in about six minutes on the first nap, but could not fall asleep on the others.

Based on all the available data, I felt that Miss B had insomnia associated with the delayed sleep phase syndrome, aggravated by poor sleep hygiene. We agreed to six weekly one-hour sessions.

During the first session, we talked mainly about sleep hygiene. Miss B was asked to cut her bedtime to seven hours and decided that she would do this from 1 A.M. to 8 A.M. I stressed that regular arousal at 8 A.M. was crucial. I also insisted on a decrease to one beer per night, to be taken at least five hours before her bedtime.

Because of the delayed sleep phase syndrome, I decided to start light therapy by having Miss B exposed to bright light for at least one hour shortly after getting up, from 8:30 A.M. to 9:30 A.M. Miss B was given a bright-light box and instructed in its use. Because this therapy is extensively explained in Chapter Twelve by Dr. Rosenberg, I will not describe it here. I also asked Miss B to keep a sleep log.

On the second session, it became clear that Miss B had not followed my recommendations. She felt that she was simply too tired to get up at 8 A.M. Three times she had used the light box, but after 11 A.M., and she had not sat in front of it for more than 15 or 20 minutes. There had been a fight with the boyfriend, and alcohol consumption had increased. I reexplained the reasons for my recommendations, and we discussed how she might get herself up around 8 A.M. Finally, Miss B decided to involve her parents, who might come over, wake her up, and get her in front of the light box, where she could eat breakfast and read.

At the next session, there was no progress. There had been a number of angry exchanges between her parents when they came over at 8 A.M. to enforce the regular sleep/wake rhythm and initiate light therapy. Even on the days when they had been successful in getting her up and in front of the light box, Miss B simply had returned to bed as soon as they left the apartment. Miss B could not see how simply sitting in front of a "stupid light box" could do anything for her inability to fall asleep at night.

I switched to relaxation therapy, trying to teach Miss B abdominal breathing. She became quite relaxed and actually fell asleep toward the end of the first half-hour training session. However, she disliked the focus on breathing because she claimed it caused a stinging sensation in her nose. She could not see the point of that. Nevertheless, by the end of the hour she agreed to practice for one-half hour each evening.

When it became clear during the following hour that Miss B had not practiced because, she claimed, it was close to the school midterm and she had no time, I tried to explore what was going on. Maybe this was not a good time to work on her insomnia? I asked what she had expected from the treatment and how she saw her continuous lack of carrying through with suggestions made in the therapy hour. I suggested that maybe we should wait for a time when she was less preoccupied with school and boyfriend.

Miss B did not see how she had frustrated the behavioral recommendations. She had tried each, but they were simply too hard, in her judgment. There was a tremendous sense of entitlement. Although never clearly expressed, Miss B seemed to feel that because she had been crippled by the accident at age 14, I owed her improved sleep and that I simply had not yet suggested a proper set of recommendations that she could follow.

The question of medication came up. Miss B wanted prescriptions for both hypnotics and stimulants to make her able to sleep when she wanted and to be awake when she wanted. I declined.

By the end of the hour, Miss B begged me to continue with treatment. She felt that relaxation therapy had helped her a little. I reinforced the abdominal breathing technique that I had taught her previously and asked her to practice this method once a day in the early evening. I gave her a form on which she should keep track of the times she did the relaxation training. She promised faithfully to do it.

At our final session, Miss B had forgotten the sheet but admitted that she had only practiced once for about ten minutes. After some nondirective exploration, trying to clarify what she herself had wanted and expected from these sessions, I told her that I would agree to see her again, but only after she had practiced relaxation for at least six half-hour periods. As soon as that happened, she was to send me her filled-out relaxation form, and I would schedule an appointment within the week.

I never saw Miss B again. She called about two weeks later, saying that she had heard of a hypnotist who could achieve the same relaxation effects without her having to practice exercises. She also claimed that all our discussions had really helped and that she now was sleeping considerably better. I doubted it.

What had gone wrong? It would be easy to simply blame Miss B's lack of motivation or her laziness. Nevertheless, she faithfully came to the scheduled sessions and seemed to want to continue. It seems more likely that she needed continued support and counseling on issues that went much deeper than her inability to sleep. In retrospect, I was simply not willing to provide that kind of long-term therapy. Hence, my rather authoritarian termination of the relationship, shifting the blame onto her.

It is not easy to follow behavioral programs. It is hard, for example, to get up at a predetermined time when you are exhausted from lack of sleep. Not everyone is a good candidate for this; not everyone can strive for a goal that might be achieved only with pain and only at some future time. It also takes self-confidence to expect that one can achieve success.

Overall, I see sleep hygiene advice, relaxation training, and some cognitive restructuring as front-line first defenses against insomnia. Many people can make amazing progress in their sleep disturbance with very few sessions, and they do not need any further work. For others, especially for those who deny or repress significant psychological stress, it is often a first step in the right direction, designed to build confidence, self-esteem, and the beginnings of a trusting relationship with the therapist that later might lead to further explorations of more complex issues.

Peter J. Hauri he received his Ph.D. in clinical psychology from the University of Chicago in 1966 with a dissertation on "The Effects of Evening Activity on Subsequent Sleep and Dreams." Subsequently, he worked at the DeWitt State

Hospital in Auborn, California (1966–1968) and at the University of Virginia Sleep Disorders Center (1968–1971) before moving to the Dartmouth Medical School in Hanover, New Hampshire. There, in 1972, he opened one of the first sleep disorders centers. Since 1988, he has been director of the Insomnia Program at the Mayo Sleep Disorders Center, where he sees an average of two new insomnia patients per day.

Dr. Hauri has done research on sleep and on insomnia since 1961, mainly studying nonpharmacological treatment approaches. He is the author of *The Sleep Disorders*, which serves as the introduction to sleep disorders for most physicians. In 1990, together with Shirley Linde, he coauthored *No More Sleepless Nights*, a self-help book for patients with insomnia. Dr. Hauri is the recipient of the 1989 Kleitman Award, given annually for outstanding service to the field.

RECOMMENDED READINGS

Davis, M., Eshelman, E. R., McKay, M. (1988). *The relaxation and stress reduction workbook*. Oakland, CA: New Harbinger Publications.
  A self-help book that summarizes the available techniques in this area.
McKay, M., Davis, M., Fanning, P. (1981). *Thoughts and feelings*. Richmond, CA: New Harbinger Publications.
  A workbook for the layman that reviews many cognitive strategies useful in the treatment of insomnia.
Meichenbaum, D. (1977). *Cognitive–behavior modification, an integrative approach*. New York: Plenum Press.
  A classic in the field of cognitive therapy by one of the most influential of clinical psychologists currently living in the United States.

REFERENCES

Adamson, J., & Burdick, J. A. (1973). Sleep of dry alcoholics. *Archives of General Psychiatry, 28,* 146–149.
Beck, A. (1970). Cognitive therapy: Nature and relation to behavior therapy. *Behavior Therapy, 1,* 184–200.
Borkovec, T. D., & Fowles, D. C. (1973). A controlled investigation of the effects of progressive and hypnotic relaxation on insomnia. *Journal of Abnormal Psychology, 82,* 153–158.
Coursey, R. D., Frankel, B. L., Gaarder, K. R., and Mott, D. E. (1980). A comparison of relaxation techniques with electrosleep therapy for chronic, sleep-onset insomnia, a sleep-EEG study. *Biofeedback and Self-Regulation, 5,* 57–73.
Crisp, A. H., & Stonehill, E. (1973). Aspects of the relationship between sleep and nutrition: A study of 375 psychiatric outpatients. *British Journal of Psychiatry, 122,* 379–394.
Czeisler, C. A., Rios, C. O., Sanchez, R., Brown, E. N., Richardson, G. S., Ronda, V. M., & Rogacz, S. (1986). Phase advance and reduction in amplitude of the endogenous circadian oscillator correspond with systematic changes in sleep-wake habits and daytime functioning in the elderly (Abstract). *Sleep Research, 15,* 268.
Ellis, A. (1975). *A new guide to rational living*. North Hollywood, CA: Wilshire Books.

Fara, J. W., Rubinstein, E. H., Sonnenschein, R. R. (1969). Visceral and behavioral responses to intraduodenal fat. *Science, 166,* 110–111.

Hauri, P. (1977). *The sleep disorders. Current concepts.* Kalamazoo, MI: Scope Publications, Upjohn.

Hauri, P. (1981). Treating psychophysiologic insomnia with biofeedback. *Archives of General Psychiatry, 38,* 752–758.

Hauri, P., & Linde, S. (1990). *No more sleepless nights.* New York: Wiley.

Hauri, P., Percy, L., Hellekson, C., Hartmann, E., & Russ, D. (1982). The treatment of psychophysiologic insomnia with biofeedback: A replication study. *Biofeedback and Self-Regulation, 7,* 223–235.

Horne, J. A., & Reid, A. J. (1985). Night-time sleep EEG changes following body heating in a warm bath. *Electroencephalography and Clinical Neurophysiology, 60,* 154–157.

Horne, J. A., & Staff, L. H. E. (1983). Exercise and sleep: Body-heating effects. *Sleep, 6,* 36–46.

Jacobs, B. L., & McGinty, D. J. (1971). Effects of food deprivation on sleep and wakefulness in the rat. *Experimental Neurology, 30,* 212–222.

Karacan, I., Thornby, J. I., Anch, A. M., *et al.* (1976). Dose-related sleep disturbances induced by coffee and caffeine. *Clinical Pharmacology & Therapeutics, 20,* 682–689.

Lack, L., Kalucy, R., & Balfour, R. (1988). Insomniacs have less decrease of body temperature following sleep onset (Abstract). *Sleep Research, 17,* 209.

Meichenbaum, D. (1977). *Cognitive–behavior modification.* New York: Plenum Press.

Merlotti, L., Roehrs, T., Zorick, F., Stepanski, E., Russo, L., & Roth, T. (1988). Rebound insomnia, duration of administration, and individual differences. *Sleep Research, 17,* 52.

Nicassio, P. M., Boylan, M. B., & McCabe, T. G. (1982). Progressive relaxation, EMG biofeedback and biofeedback placebo in the treatment of sleep-onset insomnia. *British Journal of Medical Psychology, 55,* 159–166.

Rundell, O. H., Lester, B. K., Griffiths, W. J., and Williams, H. L. (1972). Alcohol and sleep in young adults. *Psychopharmacologia, 26,* 201–218.

Southwell, P. R., Evans, C. R., Hunt, J. N. (1972). Effect of a hot milk drink on movements during sleep. *British Medical Journal, 2,* 429–431.

Williams, R. L., Karacan, I., & Hursch, C. J. (1974). *Electroencephalography (EEG) of human sleep: Clinical application.* New York: Wiley.

Woolfolk, R. L., Carr-Kaffashan, L., McNulty, T. F., and Lehrer, P. M. (1976). Meditation training as a treatment for insomnia. *Behavioral Therapy, 7,* 359–365.

Part Two

Psychotherapeutic Techniques and Pharmacotherapy

In Part Two, we review the more traditional approaches to insomnia that, in one form or another, have been with us much longer than the behavioral approaches.

The thorny issue of psychotherapy for insomniacs is explored in Chapters Six and Seven. Zarcone describes how a clinician would go about the task of deciding which insomniac should be referred for psychotherapy and which insomniac is unlikely to profit from such an experience. Second, his chapter describes different kinds of psychotherapy, including psychoanalysis, psychoanalytic psychotherapy, ego-supportive psychotherapy, time-limited dynamic therapy, and *Gestalt* therapy. The author warns against referring patients to unknown therapists practicing unknown brands of therapy, but he recommends family and group therapy for those patients whose stressors appear to lie in that direction.

While Zarcone deals mainly with longer-term therapy, Borson discusses the use of short-term, intensive therapy in the treatment of insomnia. Chronic insomnia is seen as a symptom of a breakdown in coping and in adaptation. Emotional arousal is seen as being precipitated by unexamined, unresolved emotional conflicts. The goal of therapy, in Borson's view, is to help determine the nature of these conflicts, to correct misperceptions, and to encourage a resolution of the conflict. Psychotherapy of insomnia needs to proceed fairly rapidly, according to Borson, mainly because insomniacs are typically not psychological-minded.

One might wonder why a chapter on pharmacotherapy is included in a book that emphasizes primarily behavioral and psychological interventions. However, pharmacotherapy is still the most widely used approach to insomnia, and benzodiazepine medications have established efficacy in the short-term treatment of many insomnias. However, tolerance may develop with chronic administration, and the benefits must be weighed against potential side effects, such as memory impairment, daytime sedation, and morning "hangover." In those cases where hypnotics are to be used, care should be taken to select the proper drug and dosage to suit both the individual patient and the type of sleep problem. Hypnotics vary in the onset and duration of their effects and in their metabolism. Successful treatment will also depend on giving the patient proper instructions regarding use of the medication. According to Stepanski *et al.*, any escalation of dosage by the patient is unacceptable and an indication that other, drug-free therapies should be considered.

CHAPTER SIX

Insomnia
Psychotherapy or Not?

VINCENT P. ZARCONE, JR.

> Is there such a thing as "expert judgment" about the genuineness of expressions of feeling?—Even here, there are those whose judgment is "better" and those whose judgment is "worse."
> Corrector prognoses will generally issue from the judgments of those with better knowledge of mankind.
> Can one learn this knowledge: Yes; some can. Not, however, by taking a course in it, but through *"experience."*—Can someone else be a man's teacher in this? Certainly. From time to time he gives him the right *tip*—This is what "learning" and "teaching" are like here.—What one acquires here is not a technique; one learns correct judgments. There are also rules, but they do not form a system, and only experienced people can apply them right.
> —Wittgenstein, 1953

INTRODUCTION

As can be seen from the above quotation, psychotherapy can be learned by giving the right tips, just as a craft is learned. The practitioner develops

---

Vincent P. Zarcone, Jr. • Palo Alto VA Medical Center, Palo Alto, California 94304 and Department of Psychiatry, Stanford University, School of Medicine, Stanford, California 94304.

a knack for understanding people and the interventions necessary to persuade them to alter their thoughts, feelings, and behaviors. Probably, referral for psychotherapy is also a craft, for which it takes great experience to develop expertise.

At the outset, those who deal with sleep disorders have to realize that the decision to refer clients for psychotherapy is not made using the same sort of scientific, logical deductions with which the diagnoses of sleep disorders are made. Rather, to select referrals for psychotherapy properly, one must either have had the experience of doing psychotherapy, preferably several different styles, or have colleagues with whom one interacts frequently enough to understand their thinking about the characteristics of patients who are candidates for psychotherapy.

However, before the referral is considered, a number of steps must be taken. These are rather obvious and are most often well known. They are, of course, the steps in the process of arriving at a sleep disorders diagnosis, and the secondary diagnoses which can be, and frequently are, associated with insomnia diagnoses. Insomnia is not a monolithic entity, as is well known after two decades of work on the problem. The insomnia complaint, as has been stated countless times in many educational forums since the development of sleep disorders medicine in the early 1970s, is a complaint. Period. As a complaint, it is the first step in the exploration of the syndrome or syndromes that underlie it. Therefore, the standard approach is medical, deductive logic with the use of the history, tests, and the differential diagnosis to finally arrive at a diagnosis and ancillary diagnoses of complications or associated syndromes. During this approach to the insomnia complainer, the practitioner also evaluates the possibility that psychotherapy will benefit the patient.

THE DIFFERENTIAL DIAGNOSIS OF THE INSOMNIA COMPLAINT

Using this approach to the patient, psychotherapy will almost invariably be an adjunct to another type of therapeutic approach. In other words, the first rule is to consider psychotherapy toward the end of the evaluation and not toward the beginning. The question is, "What role, if any, is psychotherapy going to play in the treatment of the patient?" It is a rare insomnia complainer indeed who will respond to psychotherapy as the only treatment.

This is a conservative approach. It is obvious that a patient should not be referred for psychotherapy if he or she is suffering from caffeinism. It is also obvious that a patient with sleep apnea syndrome and a secondary depression—even a severe, suicidal depression—cannot be expected to benefit from psychotherapy as the sole treatment. Nor is it economically feasible or wise to refer a patient with a myriad of sleep hygiene problems for psychotherapy without first taking the simple step of educating the patient. If, in the evaluation in the sleep lab, a patient is found to have an insomnia complaint without objective findings, and is also noted to be a severely hypochondriacal borderline personality, then treatment with hypnotics or insight-oriented psychotherapy is probably not indicated. Rather, what is needed is consultation with a psychiatrist experienced in the treatment of the borderline personality disorder. Similarly, in the evaluation of a patient for whom the final diagnosis is fibromyalgial syndrome, referral for psychotherapy may or may not be indicated. If the patient has a severe, long-term disorder which has incapacitated him or her, then referral for family, couples, or brief insight-oriented psychotherapy will probably not be enough. What is needed in this case is a program of behavior modification designed to help the patient cope with a chronic disease. Additionally, a patient who has had a long-term dependence on barbiturates will not profit from psychotherapy until the drug dependency issue has been dealt with. Finally, conditioned insomnia responds to behavior modification and may or may not leave a residue of psychoneurotic problems which need to be addressed in psychotherapy.

The diagnostic procedures that lead to the decision to recommend psychotherapy then begin with the standard evaluation in the sleep disorders clinic. In turn, this begins with a structured or unstructured interview to elicit all the information necessary to consider the differential diagnosis of insomnia. That is, one evaluates sleep hygiene, circadian rhythm disorders, conditioned insomnia, major and minor mood disorder, periodic leg movements, sleep apnea syndrome, illicit drug dependency and dependency on or abuse of caffeine, nicotine, or alcohol, and the presence of rare central physiological abnormalities that may, in fact, underlie the complaint. These latter, which can only be diagnosed with polysomnograms, are probably the only (and extremely rare) indications for the chronic prescription of hypnotics. (Although there are no follow-up studies to indicate effectiveness.) They include interruptions from rapid-eye-movement (REM) sleep, the REM behavior disorder, alpha/delta sleep as part of the fibromyositis syndrome, K-alpha arousals, and other abnormalities found on the polysomnogram, such as very frequent and short body movements that lead to arousal. It is mandatory to go through the steps of ruling out (or in) all these diagnoses because treatment obviously depends on the diagnosis.

INDICATIONS FOR REFERRAL FOR PSYCHOTHERAPY

For about 15 years, the American Sleep Disorders Association (Rochester, Minnesota 55902) has recommended the use of carefully controlled trials of hypnotic medication as an adjunct for two conditions. These two conditions are also the two most common ones that will result in referral of the patient for psychotherapy. One condition is conditioned insomnia, which may complicate an accompanying disorder, e.g., generalized anxiety disorder or chronic dysthymia. The second condition is an insomnia complaint associated with psychiatric conditions, e.g., syndromes such as generalized anxiety disorder or chronic dysthymia. Once the differential diagnostic process has resulted in a consideration of these disorders, then consideration of referral for psychotherapy should be mandatory. The practitioner should remember that mood disorders are extremely prevalent in our society. Conditioned insomnia can arise and become an entity which has a life and subsequent course of its own during an episode of major or minor depressive disorder. Conditioned insomnia can also be seen in patients with DSM-IIIR* Axis II disorders, perhaps most commonly, histrionic, narcissistic, and avoidant and dependent disorders. Initially, conditioned insomnia has to be treated using behavior modification. However, if the patient has conditioned insomnia and a psychiatric syndrome, then the evaluation for psychotherapy should proceed either concurrently or toward the end of treatment of the conditioned insomnia with behavior modification. The evaluation should proceed particularly in those cases of conditioned DIMS[†] which wax and wane with an associated Axis I disorder. Conditioned insomnia alone is not an indication for psychotherapy.

This brings the diagnostic treatment evaluation process to the point where the practitioner considers the cost/benefit ratio of psychotherapy, i.e., the actual referral itself.

GENERAL CONSIDERATIONS IN REFERRAL FOR PSYCHOTHERAPY

There are several general issues in the evaluation of any patient for psychotherapy. The first is motivation and economic considerations. The patient has to have some desire to at least explore the benefit of psycho-

---

*Diagnostic and Statistical Manual III R.
†Disorders of initiating and maintaining sleep.

therapy, and he must have some means of paying for it. Next is the general and verbal intelligence of the patient. During the history gathering necessary for a sleep disorders diagnosis, the general and verbal intelligence and educational status of the patient can be ascertained. Patients probably have to have verbal intelligence consistent with college-level work to benefit from psychoanalysis or psychoanalytic psychotherapy.

A certain amount of psychological sophistication is a prerequisite for benefit from psychotherapy. The history of prior experience with psychotherapy is of obvious importance. If the patient understood the process of psychotherapy, it is a good sign that he or she will be able to benefit from it again. A history of conversations with friends, ministers, or family members can also be used to ascertain the psychological sophistication of the patient. If those conversations resulted in emotional learning which was helpful to the patient, then the patient has a better prognosis for benefit in psychotherapy. Similarly, if the patient understands, or can be educated quickly to understand, the basic mechanisms of behavior modification—for instance, the interposition of a relaxation response between conditioned stimuli and conditioned response—then that is evidence for some degree of psychological sophistication that will be of benefit in psychotherapy. More general signs of sophistication include the depth of the answer to the question "Why do you think you are the way you are?" That question, which is also very useful to rule out schizophrenic conceptual disorganization, can be answered with a wide range of psychological insight. The answer "I don't know" or "I've never thought about it" is not a good sign. Familiarity with lay language psychological models and the ability to describe character are also good signs of sophistication; if a patient has not read a novel in the 10 or 15 years since college, then he or she may not be a good candidate. More specific evidence of psychological sophistication is addressed in the next section. The various theoretical bases for types of psychotherapy can be presented to the patient during the process of explaining the styles of the several therapists to whom the patient could be referred.

Another and very important considerations is the ego strength or the competence of the personality to withstand strong emotion or confusing thought processes. If the patient has an adequate or strong occupational identity, that means, by definition, that he or she is able to withstand some of the emotional turmoil that is part of any occupation. Also, by definition, the patient is able to form a working alliance with co-workers (unless the occupation requires social isolation). Another general indicator of ego strength is supportive relationships within the family and within the patient's circle of friends. Another is constructive leisure time activities. Spiritual or religious affiliation is still another general indicator. More specific examples of ego strength for particular forms of psychotherapy are given in the next section.

SPECIFIC PSYCHOTHERAPY RECOMMENDATIONS

The first consideration, although the least likely, is classical psychoanalysis. This means that the patient will be treated "on the couch" four or five times a week for 50 minutes per session at considerable expense. The patient obviously has to have above-average verbal intelligence and general signs of psychological sophistication and ego strength. More specific indicators of the latter two requisites can be obtained while describing psychoanalysis to the patient.

The modern clinical psychoanalytic approach depends on careful confrontation, clarification, interpretation, and working through of structures within the psyche. Those structures are sets of complexes of thoughts and feelings that have been elaborated during the lifetime of the patient and "transferred" from relationship to relationship, from infancy into adult life. In Greenson's (1967) explanation of psychoanalysis, the patient considers core conflicts as they are assessed in four areas. The first area is childhood, the second everyday life, the third, crisis situations; and the fourth, transference neurosis. The patient should be able to understand the basic notion of transference if he or she is to be referred for this form of psychotherapy. Transference simply means the transfer of elements of a core conflict into current relationships, the most important of which is the relationship with the analyst. This *is* the most important because it allows the patient to explore his or her perceptual distortions—that is, the patient's tendency to generalize, delete, and actively distort information in a current relationship in which there are strong emotions.

Classical psychoanalytic technique is summarized well by Greenson (1967). His book is still a classic text, in wide usage. Perhaps it is characterized best in the description of the analysis of resistance which is the key element in the resolution of the transference neurosis. Resistance is an opportunity to undo a lifetime of maladaptive work of the patient's ego, i.e., all that is repressed because of core conflicts:

> Although the patient suffering from a neurosis enters psychoanalytic treatment with the conscious motive of wanting to change, there are unconscious forces within him which oppose change, which defend the neurosis and the *status quo*. These forces oppose the procedures and processes of treatment and are called the *resistances*. Resistances stem from those same defensive forces of the ego which form part of the neurotic conflict. In the course of treatment the patient will repeat all the different forms and varieties of defensive maneuvers that he used in his past life. The analysis of the resistances is one of the

cornerstones of psychoanalytic technique. Since resistance is a manifestation of the defensive and distorting function of the ego, it is resistance which psychoanalytic technique attempts to analyze first. Insight can be effective only if the patient is able to establish and maintain a reasonable ego. Resistances interfere with the reasonable ego and have to be analyzed before any other analytic work can be done with success. (26–27).

The analysis of transference neurosis requires that the patient be able to regress and be able to experience strong emotion "on the couch." He or she has to be able to withstand the "dementia of resistance," which is a kind of confused, non-goal-directed thinking characterized by loosening of associations. In effect, the patient has to be able to withstand an almost or nearly psychotic regression on the couch and then, at the end of 50 minutes, get up and go back to work.

Also, he or she has to be able to obey another primary injunction of psychoanalysis: he or she must avoid acting out the transference by displacement. This means that the patient should be able to keep current relationships and work stable during the analysis. Major decisions have to be avoided. Otherwise, the patient may find himself misinterpreting the reasons for everyday life decisions because strong emotions are being stirred up in the transference. Withstanding analytic regression and avoiding acting out are a rough definition of ego strength as manifest in the psychoanalytic setting.

Another model of therapy is psychoanalytic psychotherapy. The same general considerations are first entertained, and then the patient's ego strength and psychological sophistication are evaluated in a similar way. Probably less ego strength is required for this form of psychoanalytic therapy *if* the therapist is highly skilled and experienced. The patient will be seen once or twice a week for two to three years; the regression and emotionality can be quite intense because the therapist will, in fact, confront and clarify in a way that deepens the transference neurosis as rapidly as possible. However, he or she will also control the level of it and use the strengths of the patient during the sessions so that the intensity is controlled. The less frequent sessions also result in a shallower transference. Not as much analytic work can be done, but it is often enough, particularly if the core conflicts are experienced most intensely in a relatively circumscribed area of the patient's life.

Ego-supportive psychotherapy based on the psychoanalytic model or the neo-Freudian interpersonal model—for instance, that of Adler, Harry Stack Sullivan or Rogers—is quite different from the first two forms of psychotherapy. It involves a play on the strength of the individual. That is, the mature coping strategies, the positive interpersonal relationships and helpful environmental influences are clarified and integrated. Transference issues are avoided if negative and exploited when positive. This form of therapy is more likely to be used in conjunction with psychopharmacological interventions. It can play an important part in the treatment of major or minor depressive disorders and of Axis II disorders. In the latter case, it may have to be done in conjunction with skills training in groups, attendance at day hospital, and so forth, depending on the severity of the personality disorder. It is the bread and butter of any therapist's practice.

The outcome statistics of all three forms of therapy covered to this point are somewhat preliminary. It is a tragedy of American psychiatry that we do not decisively know the effectiveness of these three forms of psychotherapy. If the patient wants information on effectiveness of psychotherapy, one can refer to the Smith, Glass, and Miller review (cited in Kales & Kales, 1984, p. 219):

> Smith, Glass and Miller reviewed 475 studies of psychotherapy that included approximately 25,000 patients. They found that persons who received therapy were better off in terms of symptom reduction and global improvement than 85 percent of persons who did not receive treatment. Other studies show that psychotherapy results in monetary savings in medical treatment for chronic diseases, as well as a decreased utilization of other medical services.
>
> A review of studies evaluating the predictors of psychotherapeutic outcome has shown that certain factors are associated with improvement . . . *Therapists' traits associated with improvement are level of experience, attitudes, interest patterns, empathy, and feeling of similarity between therapist and patient.* [Italics mine.] When treatment factors are considered, the number of sessions is a more powerful predictor of improvement that the type of therapy, and a combination of individual and group psychotherapy is more effective than one or the other alone.

For contrast with these outcome statistics Miller, Norman, and Keitner (1989) demonstrated significant increase in remissions—68 percent versus 33 percent—in those major depressive disorder patients who received cognitive-behavior therapy in addition to standard treatment with milieu, medication, and management sessions.

The next commonly encountered form of psychotherapy is time-limited, dynamic psychotherapy on the model of Strupp and Bender (1984). In this form of therapy, the psychological sophistication and ego strength of the patient have to be greater than in the first two; basically, this form is reserved for the mild—to moderately anxiously depressed patient who has trouble with social relationships [the 2-7-0 profile on the Minnesota Multiphasic Inventory (MMPI)] and is free of the major Axis I syndromes and also has little or no evidence of serious Axis II disorder. These patients may have had major or minor depressive disorders; it is probably contraindicated to initiate time-limited dynamic psychotherapy without medication in any patient who is experiencing a major depressive disorder episode, and certainly in any patient who bears any evidence of a schizophrenic episode. Patients with mild personality disorders are likely candidates if they have sufficient ego strength and psychological sophistication to engage a therapist in this form of therapy.

In this therapy style, there is a massive, intensive manipulation of countertransference and transference to deepen the transference neurosis rapidly, as the number of sessions is limited from 18 to 20. The tendency to regress and experience hostile reactions in the midst of these analyses of transference is remarkable. Although Strupp and Bender (1984) have initiated a program of research to explore the effectiveness of time-limited, dynamic psychotherapy, there is no evidence that this mode of therapy is effective.

Next is Gestalt therapy, an outgrowth of psychoanalytic psychotherapy that has taken on a life of its own. Fritz Perls modified the psychoanalytic approach in the 1950s partly because of the practical reasons involving great expense and lengthy treatment needed and partly because of his disillusionment with the psychogenetic model on which psychoanalysis is based (Perls, Hefferline, & Goodman, 1951). Perls sought a more open-ended, interpersonal, here-and-now systems approach that paid considerable attention to behaviors manifested in each session. The three Gestalt techniques of psychodrama, shuttling, and confusion can be explained to a sophisticated patient using examples of role playing or speaking to an empty chair; people important in the development of the patient can be brought into the therapy in an active, dramatic way by the Gestalt therapist. The issue of transference can be "addressed" by bringing in significant figures into role plays; however, there is no development of a transference neurosis. Rather, the current relationships of the individual are more intensely focused on than in the psychoanalytic therapies. The patient's ability to learn in Gestalt session is somewhat more dependent on his dramatic flair and his ability to rather immediately become aware of his feeling states, body sensations, and behaviors as they impact on others. *Gestalt* therapy requires a considerable degree of ego strength and sophistication on the part of the patient, much more than does ego-supportive psychotherapy—probably equal to that required for psychoanalysis. However, it is much less time consuming and expensive.

The derivatives of Gestalt therapy, as practiced, for instance, at the Mental Research Institute in Palo Alto, California, by Virginia Satir, emphasis the language of the Gestalt therapy process as well as the three basic techniques. The patient can be brought to an understanding of the goal of this more language-oriented Gestalt therapy by an explanation of statements that are well-formed in therapy. The goal of Satir and her trainees is to reframe the experiences of the individual in the here-and-now by using descriptions free of deletions, distortions, and generalizations.

For instance, if a patient says, "They always make me do it," the patient is generalizing with words such as "they" and "always," the patient is distorting with the use of the logical operator of necessity, which is "make," and the patient is deleting when using the word "it." The patient is brought to an awareness of his characteristic ways of interacting with others which include his own body sensations, postures, facial expressions, tone of voice, and the effects of those on the other person. This produces a state of confusion in which the therapist asks repeatedly, "What are you going to do differently now that you have experienced yourself operating in this style?" It does require a considerable psychological sophistication to understand and to learn from this intervention.

As Perls would say, if you want to engage in mutually gratifying actions with another person, then you have to see your way clear through a huge collection of memories and fantasies between the two of you. These sources of confusion are repeatedly presented to the patient as therapeutic *opportunities*. Using this approach, the patient is challenged to inhibit impulses and clarify emotions and motives while emotional.

This approach almost invariably results in some regression and, by definition, it uses confusion and a temporary lack of goal-directed thinking as an opportunity to learn a new style of interaction with other people. Gestalt therapy was first developed with anxious, depressed patients with obsessive/compulsive features. They were dramatically "broken down" by the techniques, but they had the ego strength to enjoy the loss of some of their distortions. The approach is still ideally suited to such patients.

Gestalt therapy is NOT indicated for patients with moderate or severe Axis II disorders, *unless* they are in environments in which they have external controls.

The recommendation of individual psychotherapeutic techniques further afield than Gestalt therapy requires that the practitioner become *very* familiar with the particular therapist who uses them. In general, that means that the educational background, experience, and prior supervision of the therapist has to be known personally to the referring practitioner. That is a tall, but necessary, order. Recently, the American Psychiatric Association published a treatment manual whose editor, T. Byron Carasieu, warns that "non-physician therapists who can't prescribe medication tend to improvise therapeutic acrobatics that may not be appropriate" (Crawford, 1989). If one refers a patient to a therapist who is practicing a nonstandard form of psychotherapy, one has a moral and probably legal responsibility to ensure that the practitioner is not a "quack." In my experience, there are many people who qualify for that label, and they have to be avoided.

It is probably going to become easier to avoid referrals to untrained therapists. Well-trained, supervised social workers, for example, can do 35 hours per week of insight-oriented and ego-supportive psychotherapy for salaries now affordable to public and private agencies.

Group psychotherapy is certainly indicated, both as an adjunct and as a primary form of therapy, in anxious, depressed, socially maladapted patients who are also judged to be appropriate for the other kinds of therapy mentioned earlier. Group therapy has the added benefit that the group's cohesiveness and support can be instrumental in aiding the patient during periods in which his own ego strength and psychological sophistication could not carry him in individual therapy. The self-esteem resulting from identification with recovering group members is another extremely important benefit of this form of therapy (Yalom, 1970).

Finally, marriage and family counseling should always be considered; most often, the indications are obvious if psychosocial stressors from family life are prominent in the history. Again, this can be an adjunct to therapy or the sole form of therapy for a patient who meets the requirements for the other therapies listed earlier. The psychological sophistication and competence of the patient for this type of therapy can be judged during an explanation of one or the other of the theories that underlie the approach. For instance, an example could be made using Minuchin's (1974) theory of boundaries between parents and children and the necessity for a supportive relationship between the parents, which is at least some of the time exclusive of the child. If the patient brightens when she or he hears this explanation of how family therapy issues can be explored, then the patient probably has enough sophistication to benefit from the therapy. In contrast, if the patient adamantly maintains that the childrens' misbehavior is his wife's problem, he may not benefit. Again, it is the responsibility of the referring specialist to ensure that the family or couples therapy is done by someone licensed in, trained in, and familiar with specific techniques. Familiarity with the textbooks in the field can be ascertained in conversation with the therapist both at initial referral and at follow-up.

The goal of the referral for all these interventions is a three- to six-month trial (and, in the case of short-term therapy, three to four sessions).

In summary, it is important to first determine the indication for psychotherapy, the general characteristics that will allow the patient to benefit, and the characteristics of the different types of therapy, in order to match the patients' ego strength and psychological sophistication to one or more of the therapeutic modalities. The patient must be evaluated to determine if pharmacological treatment is indicated. Periodically, the patient should be reevaluated for the same purpose. This may make referral to an M.D. psychotherapist the easiest for the peace of mind of the practitioner.

CASE HISTORY

Ms. K was 28 years old and unmarried when she first came for a consultation. She was a college English professor and was currently unemployed because of her sleep problem. The history of the present illness was as follows: Two years prior to the initial consultation she noted severe difficulty both initiating and maintaining sleep. There was a gradual onset of the problem associated with a deepening of chronic depression. She took hypnotics, mainly triazolam. On many nights she would repeat the dose at approximately 3 A.M. Her time in bed was fairly regulated in that she attempted to sleep from 10:30 P.M. to 8 A.M. The onset of her problem occurred at a time when she was very busy. She described herself as perfectionistic and hard-driving. She was disappointed in her career because of the heavy demands of grading compositions and her disillusionment in not seeing many students improve in their abilities. She was also involved in three other extracurricular activities at the college and was teaching Sunday school. She had been bothered by difficulty and indecision in a relationship with a man to whom she feels quite close, but does not believe would marry her. Approximately six months before the consultation, she had retired, medically disabled, from her teaching job.

She noted that since infancy, she had encountered sleep problems. She tossed and turned in such a way that she banged the bed until she fell asleep. This continued until she was 13 years old. She had no history of head banging, however. From the age of 13, she had difficulty falling asleep. She napped from 30 to 60 minutes in the later afternoon. She exercised every morning for approximately one hour.

The sleep problem was unrelated to her menstrual cycle; there was no history of snoring or leg jerks.

Psychosocial History

The patient described significant difficulties in her relationship with her mother. She said that she had never felt close to her, and in her adult life, the mother and she had kept distance from each other. The mother was described as anxious and perfectionistic. The patient noted that when she and her mother would get angry at someone else, they would also get angry with themselves.

Past Medical History and Review of Systems

There was no history of thyroid disease or of diabetes. The patient had been hospitalized as a child with high fevers. Eventually, she responded to treatment with antibiotics. She was allergic to codeine.

Drug History

The patient did not use illicit drugs, did not drink coffee or cola drinks, and did not smoke or use alcoholic beverages.

Mental Status Examination

On examination, the patient was oriented and there were no signs of any cognitive impairment. She did not appear intensely sleepy, but there was some suggestion of drowsiness. The most striking finding of the interview was the fact that the patient cried several times. Her affect was entirely appropriate to her thought content, and there were a range of affects. She was able to laugh and smile during the interview. There was no psychomotor retardation, and there was no evidence of any thought disorder.

Physical Examination

The physical examination, including the neurological examination, was entirely within normal limits.

MMPI

This test showed marked elevation on the depression scale. The pattern of responses was consistent with the observation during the interview that she uses intellectual defenses, repression, and denial.

Tentative Diagnoses

1. *Periodic leg movement syndrome*, as suggested by a long history of difficulty maintaining sleep prior to the onset of depressive symptoms
2. *Insomnia* associated with psychiatric disorder
3. *Minor depressive disorder*

The evaluation was continued with a nocturnal polysomnogram, which showed a total sleep time of 418 minutes, a sleep latency of 23 minutes, and a wake time after sleep onset of 41 minutes. There was no stage 3 or stage 4 sleep. There were 169 leg movements, all of which were associated with arousal. Two episodes were associated with arousal to wake.

Subsequent Course

The patient's periodic leg movement syndrome was treated with clonazepam. She experienced moderate benefit.

She remained depressed, and she noted that many of the activities of daily living were becoming too much for her and that her episodes of depression, crying, and sadness remained much as before. The patient noted that she had talked at some length with her sister, who was also her closest friend, and had experienced some relief. She was interested in psychoanalytic psychotherapy, as explained along the lines suggested earlier. She was referred for psychotherapy in her local community, and after an initial series of supportive sessions, she entered therapy with a person she described as an "ideal therapist." She remained in therapy for three years and experienced a full remission of her depressive symptoms without any psychopharmacological intervention. She was able to choose a new career in a related field and found her relationships to be much more satisfying.

Six years after her initial consultation, Ms. K moved with her husband to another area of the country. She sought and obtained another evaluation in a sleep lab, mainly to determine whether she needed to continue the medication. Her repeat nocturnal polysomnogram, done medication free, showed roughly the same amount of disturbance attributed to periodic leg movements. Clonazepam therapy was resumed.

This patient's course points up the importance of an assessment for psychiatric syndromes that can respond to psychotherapy. The patient had many strengths and was psychologically quite sophisticated. She had already benefitted from heart-to-heart talks with her sister; she showed a pattern of responses on the MMPI which is highly consistent with a response to psychotherapy. Her interest in psychotherapy deepened upon hearing an explanation of how it might work for her, particularly in the transference of her maladaptive perceptions from her relationship with her mother to a relationship with others upon whom she was dependent in any way. Her interest in language, particularly the psychological language of nineteenth- and twentieth-century novels, was apparent. She has high verbal intelligence and readily understood the interaction between organic and psychological causes for her sleep disturbance.

Vincent P. Zarcone, Jr., is a board-certified psychiatrist who has worked at the Palo Alto VA Hospital and at the Stanford Sleep Disorders Clinic for over 20 years. Dr. Zarcone received his medical training at the University of Illinois and did his residency in Psychiatry at Stanford University. He has been on the faculty of the Department of Psychiatry at Stanford since 1967. At the Stanford Sleep Disorders Center, he specializes in the treatment of insomnia. Dr. Zarcone has evaluated and counseled over 400 patients with insomnia complaints.

Dr. Zarcone has been active in sleep research, mainly studying sleep physiology in psychopathologic states, e.g., REM sleep in schizophrenia. He has been on a number of committees of the American Sleep Disorders Association, including both nosology committees.

RECOMMENDED READINGS

Greenson, R. R. (1967). *The technique and practice of psychoanalysis.* New York: International Universities Press.
This book provides a theoretical introduction to psychodynamic psychotherapy that is classic in its clarity and elegance. It has richly detailed examples of interpretation, confrontation, clarification, and working through.

Minuchin, S. (1974). *Families and family therapy.* Cambridge, MA: Harvard University Press.
This book proceeds from the systems theory base of family therapy. It details boundaries in normal and troubled families.

Strupp, H. H., & Bender, J. L. (1984). *Psychotherapy in a new key.* New York: Basic Books.
Based on the systematic study of a new technique, this book suggests a framework for much needed clinical research.

Yalom, I. D. (1970). *The theory and practice of group psychotherapy.* New York: Basic Books.
Probably the most widely read and cited text on the subject, this book is based on objective and subjective data gathered in hundreds of hours of group psychotherapy. It describes curative factors and continues to serve as a benchmark for evaluation of group process.

REFERENCES

Crawford, M. H. (1989). Briefings. *Science 245,* 934.
Greenson, R. R. (1967). *The technique and practice of psychoanalysis.* New York: International Universities Press.
Kales, A., & Kales, J. D. (1984). Psychotherapy and behavior therapy. *The evaluation and treatment of insomnia.* New York: Oxford University Press.
Miller, I. W., Norman, W. H., & Keitner, G. I. (1989). Cognitive–behavioral treatment of depressed inpatients: Six- and twelve-month follow-up. *American Journal of Psychiatry, 146,* 1274–1279.
Minuchin, S. (1974). *Families and family therapy.* Cambridge, MA: Harvard University Press.
Perls, F., Hefferline, R. F., and Goodman, P. (1951). *Gestalt therapy.* New York: Crown Publishers/Bantam Books.
Strupp, H. H., & Bender, J. L. (1984). *Psychotherapy in a new key.* New York: Basic Books.
Wittgenstein, L. (1953). *Philosophical investigations* (3rd ed.) New York: Macmillan.
Yalom, I. D. (1970). *The theory and practice of group psychotherapy.* New York, London: Basic Books.

CHAPTER SEVEN

Short-Term Psychotherapy for Chronic Insomnia

ANDREW J. BORSON

INTRODUCTION

Can short-term psychotherapy be used to treat chronic insomnia? I believe that in many cases it can, with minimal use of behavioral or pharmacological interventions, and with complete eradication of the insomnia problem.

Since not all insomniacs benefit from short-term psychodynamically informed psychotherapy, or at least present challenges to this technique, I will also address the question of how these people can be identified early in evaluation and treatment. I will present some guidelines and suggestions concerning these questions.

My clinical training reflects a combination of psychodynamic, cognitive, and family systems therapies. I have attempted to approach the treatment of chronic insomnia from these various perspectives, and I have made particular use of cognitive therapy approaches in dealing with the perfectionistic and "disaster"-predicting people who seem to benefit most from a rationalistic approach. I have also made use of stimulus control (Bootzin & Nicassio, 1978; Lacks, 1987) and sleep restriction (Spielman, Saskin, & Thorpy, 1987), but subsume these interventions under the more general heading of "cognitive therapy" approaches for reducing anxiety about not sleeping. I have made use of family systems theory in understanding secondary-gain operations of insomnia, and particularly in developing interventions to reverse these maladaptive rewards.

Andrew J. Borson • Sleep Disorders Center, Crozer-Chester Medical Center, Chester, Pennsylvania 19013.

I have found, however, that a significant number of the insomniacs whom I treat can benefit from short-term, psychodynamically informed psychotherapy, with minimal need for structured cognitive/behavioral interventions or pharmacological interventions.

I conceptualize functional chronic insomnia as a symptom of a breakdown in coping and adaptation. This occurs initially because of a specific stress, albeit one that may not be apparent to the person at the time. However, the stress touches an underlying area of unresolved emotional conflict; therefore, the conflictual feelings may continue to create turmoil long after the precipitating stress has ended. Furthermore, if the symptom of insomnia persists long enough (several years), it may become part of the person's characterological structure, coming to seem a "normal," if unpleasant, part of life, and occurring in a seemingly random manner because of now having multiple psychological functions and meanings. This follows, essentially, from the views expressed by White (1948, 1963), MacKinnon and Michels (1971), and many others writing in a similar vein on the nature of neurotic symptom formation and assimilation of the symptom into the person's character.

From this perspective, insomnia occurs, as a symptom, because of emotional arousal precipitated by unexamined and unresolved emotional conflict. The goal of therapy, then, is to help the person determine the nature of the underlying conflicts, bring them into relief against what the person knows to be true (correct the misperceptions), and then encourage a resolution of the conflicts (which may take the form of reevaluating one's self, accepting unhappy aspects of one's past, or actively changing unsatisfying current relationships or situations). Here, I draw on therapy descriptions of Sifneos (1972, 1987), Bruch (1974), Fromm-Reichmann (1960), as well as my own psychotherapy experience treating many types of problems.

Finally, I also believe that the psychotherapy of insomnia problems, like the psychotherapy of any somatic complaint, must be effective fairly rapidly, or else the patient will be "lost" and will pursue physicalistic explanations and treatments of the problem. This is a stronger possibility with some people than with others (essentially, the so-called "psychological mindedness" of the person is at question here), but in my experience it is a factor, to some extent, in nearly all cases of insomnia. For this reason, I believe the therapist must take an active, somewhat directive approach, with continued focusing of the therapy on the problems and conflicts that underlie the insomnia symptom. Here, I take my cue from the thinking of Sifneos (1987) and others in the brief-psychotherapy movement.

I know of little research into the effectiveness of traditional or short-term "uncovering" types of therapies on insomnia. Kales and Kales (1984) report that psychotherapy, in their view, is the best treatment for chronic insomnia, but they seem to be reaching this conclusion from experience, rather than research.

Finally, I know of few discussions that attempt to set forth the patient selection factors that strongly suggest psychotherapy, or that, alternatively, may suggest other treatment approaches. I do think there are many people who will be too resistant to an "uncovering" therapy to enter into such a process, and for them, a behavioral, pharmacological, or possibly structured cognitive approach may be more useful, at least at first. I return to the question of patient selection factors and readiness in the Discussion.

METHOD

Most of my insomnia patients have been screened by a sleep medicine physician for problems such as sleep apnea and periodic leg movements, and some may have undergone polysomnography. During my initial evaluation, I am trying to categorize the person by type of insomnia diagnosis (depression/anxiety, conditioning without depression, hypochondriacal, circadian, etc.), and by what sorts of interventions are likely to work for this person based on his or her personality.

I inquire about the quality of the insomnia experience for the person—is he aware of feeling tense, frustrated, or alert (thereby suggesting significant somatized tension), or does he report feeling relaxed yet not sleepy (which, if the problem is not circadian, may suggest "la belle indifference" of an hysterical conversion symptom)? Does the person describe chronic worrying and concerns about performance (which can point to an obsessional and perfectionistic attitude, possibly with depression)? What is the focus of the worrying (which may suggest the core conflicts that are being expressed)? In the case of a person who is unaware of "worry," except for worry about not sleeping (which in my experience occurs in all insomnia patients who seek treatment), what else *might* he be worried about? Here, I make the working assumption that the focus in such a person's insomnia is a displacement from other, more disruptive and threatening, conflicts.

I inquire, for all patients, but especially for this last group, about marital and family histories, precipitating factors at the time the insomnia began, and key points in the person's life for which there are emotionally powerful memories. I also inquire about the reactions of family members to the person's insomnia, as a way of indirectly seeking information about secondary gain. Through such a comprehensive interpersonal history, the shape of the person's key conflict areas often emerges.

I use psychological testing to supplement the interview. I find that the Minnesota Multiphasic Personality Inventory (MMPI) gives quick, accurate information regarding the extent to which hypochondriacal or depressive features may be present. The Rorschach test can be helpful in revealing core emotional conflicts.

I tend to see most insomnia cases as falling along a spectrum of treatment, with straightforward "uncovering" psychotherapy at one end, and a very structured approach using behavioral, cognitive training, and strategic (and paradoxical) approaches at the other. In theory, I believe it should be possible to do a complete enough evaluation so that a specific plan and approach can be adopted at the start, although in practice, I know that this is often not the case. However, some of the factors I look for in making this determination include the following: awareness of some of the underlying emotional conflicts, worry as a key experience (rather than somatized tension or lack of concern), evidence of some degree of subjective depression or distress beyond the insomnia complaint, and a willingness to adopt a psychological framework for the problem, rather than a strictly physiological framework. Generally, also, I attempt to find out what the person was looking for—whether symptom relief or resolution of the underlying "problem." Of course, I am aware that "mere" symptom relief is often a major step toward resolving underlying problems associated with feelings of inadequacy, helplessness, and lack of control.

Once I have decided to use the "uncovering" technique, my approach involves many of the moves of typical psychotherapy: building a rapport with the person, encouraging the person to describe his significant relationships, asking questions about conflicts that are being expressed in terms of those relationships, and encouraging the person to explore the links between the conflicts and his emotional states and ruminative thoughts. As these connections are made, I encourage the patient to resolve the conflicts, making suggestions, as needed, about how that might be done. These may be interpersonal actions or, just as frequently, a matter of changing perceptions ("reframing") about past or present conflicts.

I monitor the extent to which the person is experiencing ruminative thinking when trying to sleep and keep relating that thinking back to underlying issues and unresolved conflicts. In this way, the focus of the therapy remains on the presenting problem of insomnia, and the conflicts that are getting resolved are the ones that are creating the emotional arousal that is interfering with sleep.

SUCCESSFUL CASE

At presentation, H was a 61-year-old woman who had been having difficulty with sleep initiation and maintenance for two years. She experienced ruminative thinking, somatized tension, and irritability about her sleep disturbance. Her daytime alertness was still adequate for her to perform her duties as a health care professional, but she experienced subjective anxiety and depression, as well as mild agoraphobia. There was a slight increase in appetite and no early-morning awakening; a polysomnogram that revealed normal rapid-eye-movement (REM) parameters, with reduced sleep efficiency.

H was aware of various disturbing and conflicting events that she thought might have played some part in the onset and maintenance of her insomnia. She was struggling with her disapproval and unhappiness over several decisions that her youngest, adult son had made, culminating in his denying paternity of a child that she felt was certainly his. In the evaluation, she acknowledged feeling that there was some connection between this family problem and her insomniac ruminations. At the next meeting, she was also accepting of the idea that her "personality style" was oriented toward self-criticism, perhaps excessively, and that this self-criticism, along with criticism of others, underlaid much of her nighttime thinking.

Psychological testing (Rorschach and MMPI) was suggestive of mild depression, with roots in a disturbed relationship with her mother, whom she experienced as rejecting, overly controlling, and impossible to please. This led to feelings of basic insecurity and inadequacy. H coped with these feelings by adopting a moralistic and "external" standard for judging herself and others, which approached some of the perfectionistic and controlling attitudes of her mother. This gave H a means of reducing her anxiety about her adequacy, although it still left her vulnerable to bouts of feeling inadequate, as those underlying feelings could never be resolved in this "patching over" manner.

Over the course of 26 psychotherapy sessions, it was possible to bring out the underlying self-esteem issues and to productively trace them back to their roots. This allowed a reevaluation of H's sense of personal competency and permitted her to adopt a more human, flexible standard for judging others and herself. She was less angry with her son, better able to understand some of his motivations, and able to talk to him productively about what had happened. She was less angry and disappointed in herself as a mother. She was able to see that some of her reaction to her son's denial of paternity related back to her felt sense of her mother as rejecting. Presumably, her positive transference to me as an accepting, tolerant parent figure may have helped her through this work as well.

This was followed by partial exploration of some long-standing marital problems, and by some productive work on how she handled anger toward family members. She was able to express anger and other feelings toward her husband in a less guilt-ridden way. One final issue, related to how she had developed a "caretaker" role toward an older family member, was only briefly discussed, and H indicated that she did not feel it was necessary for her to explore this relationship.

H's sleep disturbance had alleviated by the eighth session, following the point at which she started feeling differently about her son. All along, I had been asking her about the kinds of "worry" she was experiencing at night, and the general theme always seemed related to issues about her son. Her mood did not stably improve until about the twentieth session, however, which was the point at which we had also dealt with self-esteem and marital problems.

H returned six months later to talk for one session about concerns she was having about another of her children. However, these problems were not a source of depression or sleep disturbance to her, and I had the definite sense that she just wanted to "check in" with me. Over the six months, she had continued to feel well and sleep well. I have not heard from her for two years since then and presume that she continues to function well.

Some salient points about this case are the following: This woman was accepting of the idea that her insomnia had an emotional basis and was able to focus on several key areas of emotional conflict in a relatively brief period of time. She had developed a positive transference to me that suggested she was "ready" to work on these issues. We focused on issues that were most directly associated with her ruminations/"worries" and with her perceived reasons for depression, but also explored childhood family dynamics as a means of resolving self-esteem problems. H did not want to work on areas that she felt were unrelated to her subjective distress and did not appear to need to do so in order to achieve a reasonably defined "successful" outcome.

Could a behavioral approach have worked for H? Possibly, but the underlying issues associated with suppressed anger and poor self-esteem would not have surfaced and been resolved, which may have prevented the complete or long-lasting treatment of the insomnia. In addition, by treatment of the underlying issues, H's feelings of depression were also resolved, thereby solving two problems for her. Finally, the act of learning to uncover and work through emotional conflicts may help H in the future if she faces new, potentially disruptive, stresses.

I might also note that this is a woman whom I had initially seen as histrionic, and as having some secondary-gain features to her insomnia (which were dealt with indirectly in the course of resolving some of the marital problems). There was a clear emotional precipitant to her insomnia, with continuing emotional distress above and beyond the insomnia complaint. However, she could not be diagnosed as having a major depression.

Therapy was relatively focused and oriented toward reevaluation of self, increased understanding of emotional reactions, and a problem-solving approach to interpersonal conflicts.

UNSUCCESSFUL CASE

At presentation, R was a 40-year-old woman who had been having intermittent difficulty with sleep maintenance since age ten. She experienced episodic, performance-related ruminative thinking, but at other times was unaware of any specific arousing thoughts. She reported mild impairment in her daytime performance (possibly more subjective than objective) and noted that family members were aware of increased irritability on her part when her sleep suffered. She was a successful business executive, who, during the course of treatment, received a significant promotion. She denied daytime anxiety or depression, except as related to her insomnia. A polysomnogram confirmed multiple awakenings and reduced delta sleep percent, with no REM-related pathology. Previously, she had been treated with benzodiazepines and tricyclic antidepressants, with limited success.

R had no explanation for her insomnia. She acknowledged experiencing job-related stress and expressed chronic dissatisfaction with her employer, but felt there was no direct temporal relationship between increased job pressures and worsened insomnia. She described a relatively satisfying marriage, with some tension associated with one of her children, but noted that her insomnia problem had long preceded being a parent. The MMPI revealed mild anxiety and depression and some tendency toward internalizing anger. Unfortunately, the Rorschach test was not administered.

Over the course of 15 sessions, R wavered in her interest in, and acceptance of, underlying emotional conflicts as a factor in her insomnia. We were able to trace problems she had had with separation anxiety from her mother, whom she saw as an insincere, insecure woman. Further, it appeared likely that her childhood bouts of insomnia were directly related to times when she was away from her mother. However, R seemed to experience little, if any, relief in making these connections, possibly because the precipitating reasons for the insomnia were no longer significant—or because she continued to maintain a certain degree of doubt about the process of uncovering emotional conflicts.

As this historical approach failed to lead anywhere, I then went back to R's current ruminations for clues, and we started focusing on her manifest anxieties about her work performance. She was prone to "worst case" or "disaster" scenarios, which had never actually occurred, but which produced sufficient anxiety/arousal to lead to long bouts of middle-of-the-night wakefulness. As noted above, the objective evidence suggested that she actually performed quite well, but like many perfectionists, she could never convince herself that a disaster wasn't around the corner.

R was unable to make any direct connections between this fear of failure and her history, but was able to relate some of these fears and sense of inadequacy to her mother's ignoring her real accomplishments and focusing extensively on her appearance. I worked with R on reevaluating this way of looking at herself, and even went so far as to sketch out for her the beliefs she held that kept her from ever feeling competent.

At this point, R started experiencing angry feelings, not only at the way she felt "locked" into her perfectionism, but also at her mother for interfering with her developing a stronger sense of competence. At the session immediately following this realization, she came in, and announced that she had solved the problem of her insomnia—she merely had to eliminate her (single) morning cup of coffee, and her sleep would be fine. She felt pleased (and competent!) at solving her problem and at discovering that she had a "physical" reason for her insomnia after all. She did note that she had been successful in handling an interaction with her mother in a way that led her to feel less anger and guilt. With that as a final comment, she terminated treatment. While no follow-up is available, I tend to doubt that eliminating the one cup of coffee would have had a long-term effect on her sleep problems. It seems evident to me that she had a "flight into health" when the issues we were discussing became too frightening.

In reviewing this history, three years later, certain factors are apparent. First, there was no clear-cut agenda that R agreed to that related her insomnia to emotional factors. There were times when she started to accept this explanation, but most of the time, she was doubtful. Second, the evaluation was incomplete in that I could not make a reasonable guess at the start as to the psychological reasons for her insomnia. As part of this, I think I missed seeing the extent to which her insomnia had changed in its meaning to her, from a disturbing expression of emotional distress to an emblem of her feelings of incompetence. That is, her insomnia had taken on a symbolic meaning, much like a conversion symptom or an eating disorder. There were important psychological reasons for her *not* to get better, and I did not see that until it was too late.

Third, negative transference feelings were being felt and expressed, and I did not pursue these effectively. I dealt with them only on the level of confronting R's ambivalence about psychotherapy, but not on the more important level of exploring her concerns about "opening up" (and getting in touch with angry feelings) or dealing with her reactions to me as someone pressing her to give up a comfortable, if maladaptive, way of looking at herself. I spoke to these issues indirectly, but might have focused on them more intensively.

Much of therapy was spent developing a formulation and attempting to find a workable common ground. The defensive aspects of the insomnia "symptom" were not fully appreciated. It is also possible that even if a complete formulation of the problem was available at the start, R would still have resisted working on the problem at some crucial point. However, in that situation, it would have been easier to challenge her desire to "escape" more effectively, or to develop strategies that "protected" the insomnia (and the internalization of anger and feelings of incompetence it represented), until R was ready to truly change.

DISCUSSION

It is my untested assumption that short-term, "uncovering" (psychodynamically informed) psychotherapy is an effective treatment for at least certain chronic insomniacs and is the treatment of choice, because of its effectiveness, when it is possible. As my "successful" case illustrates, psychotherapy can lead to a complete cure for insomnia, as well as related mild anxiety and depression.

A comparison of the two presented cases may offer some suggestions about when psychotherapy is contraindicated, or when it must be modified with other approaches.

First, the most basic question is whether the person can accept, after the evaluation (and the ruling out of apnea, leg movements, and circadian-phase disorders), formulation of the insomnia problem as one involving emotional conflict or distress. It seems clear to me that until this basic agreement occurs, psychotherapy will be inadequate for the person. This is not to say that the person will not accept that the insomnia has an emotional basis at a later date, but it seems almost certain that without this agreement, it is wiser and more productive to attempt either a straightforward behavioral approach or a pharmacological approach.

One possible route to go, with someone who is aware of ruminative thinking, is to work on reducing the ruminative thinking through behavioral/cognitive techniques (scheduled "worry time," thought-stopping techniques, etc.) and then, if those approaches do not prove effective, ask the person to consider what might lie behind the content of the ruminations. This may open the door for a discussion of self-esteem issues, concerns about competency, and so forth.

Another key issue is whether the insomnia is only a by-product of an emotionally disturbing conflict or has become assimilated as part of the person's self-image. I know that, traditionally, sleep psychologists and psychiatrists have used the notion of conditioned arousal states to explain the continued anxiety associated with the fear of not sleeping in the long-term insomniac, but I think another way of looking at the long-term chronic insomniac is as someone for whom the "idea" of not being able to sleep has taken on symbolic meaning in how the person conceptualizes him/herself. In the case of R, it became clear in retrospect that she had bound up her feelings of incompetence in her view of herself as an insomniac, and solving her insomnia problem would mean helping her reorganize how she viewed her overall abilities and competencies, as well as how she viewed her "failure" to "control" her sleep. This is certainly psychotherapy, but of a different kind than that of the person whose insomnia is primarily due to emotional upset. The latter patient will present far less resistance to change.

Although not specifically discussed here, it is also worth considering the situation in which a person's chronic, long-term insomnia has become part of his or her image in the family. Again, this may lead to valuable insights into "secondary gain" and symptom maintenance operations that occur within the family system and may suggest interventions based on such a family dynamic formulation.

Third, it is important to keep therapy focused on problems that can be directly related to the symptom of disturbed sleep, at least in the short run. Insomniacs are suffering, and they need to see positive change in a relatively short time if they are to stick with a treatment approach. Further, it makes sense to use the presenting problems (often as expressed through the content of nighttime ruminations) to orient oneself to the most emotionally disturbing aspects of the person's conflict areas. As a counterbalance, however, it can also be useful to have a clear formulation of the person's personality dynamics as a whole before getting into therapy. This comes best, in my view, from a thorough introductory history that focuses on family relationships and problems occurring when the insomnia worsened, and through projective and objective personality testing.

Finally, the psychotherapy of chronic insomniacs can be very demanding on the skillfulness of the therapist. Convincing (demonstrating, manipulating, etc.) someone to look at psychological factors when they may see their problems as "physical" can be very challenging, but beyond that, the problems that emerge as therapy progresses can be quite difficult. Secondary-gain and negative-transference feelings can easily present roadblocks to change. These are common problems for many insomniacs, and effective interventions are needed if therapy is to keep from stalling.

Further, I suggest that the assumption be that the bulk of therapy can be completed in a relatively short period of time, approximately 20 to 30 sessions, so as to keep the therapist focused on the presenting problem of the insomnia and its associated emotional underpinnings, rather than on other problems that may emerge as therapy proceeds. If the person wants to continue in therapy to work on these other problems, that, of course, is reasonable, but a relatively focused and problem-solving approach seems essential in the initial treatment of the insomniac. This still gives time to deal with historical issues and issues related to self-esteem, but always from the perspective of the key conflicts underlying the insomnia, and with less attention to tangential issues (*cf.* Sifneos, 1987).

A. J. Borson, Sleep Psychologist at Crozer-Chester Medical Center's Sleep Disorders Center, has been treating insomnia patients for several years, using both the approach outlined here as well as more behavioral approaches, such as stimulus control and sleep restriction. Dr. Borson received his Ph.D. from the University of Pennsylvania, where he studied and worked in an environment that ranged from structural family therapy approaches at Philadelphia Child Guidance Center, to psychodynamic approaches at the Institute of Pennsylvania Hospital. Additionally, he has had extensive training in cognitive–behavioral approaches, as well as psychodynamic marital and family therapy.

RECOMMENDED READINGS

Kales, A., & Kales, J. D. (1984). *Evaluation and treatment of insomnia*. New York: Oxford University Press.
   This book focuses on common psychodynamic factors underlying chronic insomnia, as well as some of the typical resistances encountered in insomniac patients. This text is quite useful in helping a clinician develop a formulation based on underlying emotional issues, although the treatment approach advocated is different from mine and follows a more traditional psychoanalytic model.
MacKinnon, R. A., & Michels, R. (1971). *The psychiatric interview in clinical practice*. Philadelphia: Saunders.
   This is a brief textbook on understanding the psychodynamics of various personality types and symptom complaints, which can be quite valuable in orienting a therapist to the underlying emotional issues likely to be key to effective problem resolution.
Sifneos, P. E. (1987). *Short-term dynamic psychotherapy: Evaluation and technique (2nd ed.)*. New York: Plenum Press.
   This book provides an excellent model for the use of psychodynamic formulations in an active and short-term psychotherapy that focuses on helping the patient recognize and break through emotional blocks and conflicts. While

there is no direct application to insomnia, the form of treatment I describe is derived in part from the Sifneos model.

REFERENCES

Bootzin, R. R., & Nicassio, P. M. (1978). Behavioral treatments for insomnia. In M. Hersen, R. Eisler, & P. Miller (Eds.), *Progress in behavior modification (Vol. 6)*. New York: Academic Press.
Bruch, H. (1974). *Learning psychotherapy: Rationale and ground rules*. Cambridge: Harvard University Press.
Fromm-Reichmann, F. (1960). *Principles of intensive psychotherapy*. Chicago: University of Chicago Press.
Kales, A., & Kales, J. D. (1984). *Evaluation and treatment of insomnia*. New York: Oxford University Press.
Lacks, P. (1987). *Behavioral treatment for persistent insomnia*. Oxford: Pergamon Press.
MacKinnon, R. A., & Michels, R. (1971). *The psychiatric interview in clinical practice*. Philadelphia: Saunders.
Sifneos, P. E. (1972). *Short-term psychotherapy and emotional crises*. Cambridge: Harvard University Press.
Sifneos, P. E. (1987). *Short-term dynamic psychotherapy: Evaluation and technique (2nd ed.)*. New York: Plenum Press.
Spielman, A. J., Suskin, P., & Thorpy, M. J. (1987). Treatment of chronic insomnia by restriction of time in bed. *Sleep, 10*, 45–56.
White, R. W. (1948). *The abnormal personality*. New York: Ronald Press.
White, R. W. (1963). *Ego and reality in psychoanalytic theory*. New York: International Universities Press.

CHAPTER EIGHT

Pharmacotherapy of Insomnia

EDWARD J. STEPANSKI, FRANK J. ZORICK,
AND THOMAS ROTH

INTRODUCTION

For the purposes of this chapter, "hypnotic medication" is synonymous with "benzodiazepine sedative–hypnotics." In our opinion, there is almost never an indication to use an older, nonbenzodiazepine hypnotic (e.g., barbiturates, chloral hydrate, glutethimide, meprobamate) for the treatment of insomnia. In situations where depression or nonrestorative sleep syndrome (alpha–delta sleep) is present, the use of a sedating tricyclic antidepressant may be indicated. This will be discussed later.

Although it is generally agreed that the use of hypnotics is not the treatment of choice, particularly in patients with chronic insomnia, there are circumstances that warrant their use (National Institute of Mental Health, 1984). Benzodiazepines have been shown to be effective hypnotics in a number of studies with patients having chronic insomnia (Veldkamp, Straw, Metzler, & Demissianos, 1974; Perkins & Hinton, 1974; Bornstein & Cujo, 1974; Vogel, Barker, Gibbons, & Thurmond, 1976; Roth, Hartse, Saab, Piccione, & Kramer, 1980; Roehrs, Vogel, Wittig, Zorick, Paxton, Lamphere, & Roth, 1986). Decreased latency to sleep, decreased wake after sleep onset, and increased total sleep time are typical of the sleep effects reported. No tolerance is found for up to three or four weeks of chronic administration (Kales, Kales, Bixler, & Scharf, 1975). Some studies report continued efficacy and others find that tolerance develops for periods of

---

Edward J. Stepanski, Frank J. Zorick, and Thomas Roth • Sleep Disorders and Research Center, Henry Ford Hospital, Detroit, Michigan 48202.

administration longer than four weeks (Greenblatt, 1980; Moskowitz & Smiley, 1984). Daytime performance and nighttime memory have been shown to be impaired following use of hypnotics (Nicholson, 1981; Johnson & Chernik, 1982; Roehrs, Zorick, Sicklesteel, Wittig, Hartse, & Roth, 1983; Roehrs, Kribbs, Zorick, & Roth, 1986). Daytime effects occur with benzodiazepines having a long half-life, and also with short-acting drugs taken in high dosages. Anterograde amnesia has been found with hypnotic use and is more severe with higher dosages. The decision to use hypnotics, and which hypnotic to use, must consider the balance between therapeutic gains and these potential side effects.

Appropriate treatment of insomnia, whether pharmacological or behavioral, relies on an understanding of the cause of the insomnia. Particularly in chronic insomnia, a determination must be made of the extent to which the insomnia is secondary to psychiatric illness, medical illness, behavioral factors, medication effects, or a primary sleep disorder. These five areas all require specific assessment, because every patient will have multiple factors that are disturbing his or her sleep. Proper evaluation and diagnosis of the symptom is needed as the selection of a specific benzodiazepine will depend on matching the characteristics of the individual patient and the underlying etiology of the insomnia to attributes of the medication. In the case of short-term insomnia, the cause may be straightforward (e.g., situational stress, acute medical illness) and symptomatic treatment with hypnotics may be appropriate for a limited period (two to four weeks). Use of the rules described below will increase the chances of continuing improved sleep upon discontinuation. To make a diagnosis in patients with chronic insomnia (disrupted sleep for six months or longer), we interview the patient to obtain a sleep history, medical history, and psychiatric history. A brief physical examination is also given. A polysomnogram is performed only if a definite cause of the insomnia is not evident from the initial interview. A major affective illness or acute medical problem (e.g., congestive heart failure) may be present, and these conditions can then be directly treated before the sleep complaint is evaluated further. Also, there are often behavioral factors that must be addressed before additional evaluation is possible. Poor habits, such as excessive use of alcohol or caffeine, or an irregular sleep–wake schedule must be modified before a polysomnogram is appropriate. If these basic behavioral factors are improved, and sleep is still poor, then the polysomnogram is performed and a diagnosis is made. About 30 to 40 percent of patients presenting with insomnia at our center eventually receive polysomnograms. Although we may at times initiate behavioral treatment based on the interview data, we do not use hypnotics for patients with chronic insomnia unless we have a diagnosis based on polysomnographic data.

Patients with the following conditions may be likely candidates for treatment with hypnotic medications:

1. Short-term insomnia (e.g., situational stress or trauma)
2. Certain psychiatric conditions, such as anxiety disorders
3. Severe psychophysiological insomnia/childhood-onset insomnia
4. Restless legs/periodic leg movements
5. Medical conditions, pain, or medications
6. Any patient whose insomnia is refractory to other treatments (as long as there are no contraindications; see Discussion for a presentation of contraindications relevant to this approach)

Medication may be used in conjunction with behavioral treatments or may be the sole intervention in the treatment of insomnia. As behavioral treatment is discussed in detail in other chapters, we will not describe it here. We must note, however, that we always incorporate behavioral changes into any pharmacological treatment plan. Behavioral factors, relating both to sleep habits and to how the drug is used, are very important in the success of pharmacotherapy. At a minimum, we recommend behavioral monitoring with sleep diaries, especially in the early phases of treatment, and observation of sleep hygiene rules. All the sleep hygiene recommendations (e.g., avoidance of caffeine and alcohol, regular sleep–wake schedule) should be observed by all patients being treated for insomnia, regardless of the underlying cause for their insomnia. We also have specific rules for drug-taking behavior, which will be described below.

CHOICE OF MEDICATION

Practitioners should remain flexible and choose the drug that will most benefit an individual patient. Our experience has been that many physicians develop a preference for a certain benzodiazepine and use it routinely for complaints of insomnia, independent of individual differences among patients. This does not mean that a clinician need be familiar with *all* hypnotics. A practitioner should probably select a limited number of hypnotics that are representative of the different characteristics of these medications to use as the situation dictates. The differences between medications are described below. At a minimum, the clinician should be familiar with one short-acting and one long-acting drug. This strategy will allow him to gain clinical experience with the dose–response efficacy and side effect patterns of specific drugs. While many benzodiazepines are available on the market, there are a small number of differences between them which affect their benefit to different patients. The next section will review these differences.

Duration of Effect

Half-Life. The distinction between benzodiazepines that is most relevant to use for insomnia is the duration of action (see Table 1). The duration of therapeutic effect of these compounds ranges from a few hours to a few days, and this must be considered in selecting a specific drug for a patient. Continued sedation after arising in the morning may be a side effect for some or a therapeutic effect in others. For example, a 37-year-old patient with an anxiety disorder may benefit from the daytime sedation that accompanies flurazepam, 30 mg, while a 62-year-old complaining of daytime sleepiness in addition to insomnia would not. Further, the 62-year-old might experience drug buildup with chronic use to a greater extent that the younger patient. In another example, a patient who primarily complains of sleep-onset insomnia may do very well with a short-acting, rapidly absorbed compound (e.g., triazolam, 0.125 to 0.25 mg), but a patient with multiple awakenings through the night should be given a drug with an intermediate duration in order to provide peak sedation later in the sleep period.

Dosage. The duration of action of a hypnotic will also vary as a function of the dosage used. Even short-acting drugs, if given in large enough doses, will stay active the day after nighttime administration. The reasonable dosage for use in the treatment of insomnia for commonly used benzodiazepines is provided in Table 1. A smaller dose may be used, especially in older individuals or in patients who have a history of a medical disorder that affects drug metabolism (e.g., liver disease). However, larger dosages than those listed are not recommended and are typically associated with adverse effects, such as rebound insomnia and amnesia. A possible exception to this would be in the case of a patient with

Table 1. Pharmacokinetics and Dosage Range for Benzodiazepines

Generic name	Duration of action	Absorption	Recommended dosage (mg)
Alprazolam	Short	Intermediate	0.5–2.0
Chlordiazepoxide	Intermediate	Intermediate	10.0–25.0
Clorazepate	Long	Fast	7.5–15.0
Diazepam	Long	Fast	2.0–10.0
Flurazepam	Long	Intermediate	15.0–30.0
Lorazepam	Intermediate	Intermediate	0.5–2.0
Oxazepam	Intermediate	Slow	15.0–30.0
Temazepam	Intermediate	Intermediate	15.0–30.0
Triazolam	Ultrashort	Fast	0.125–0.25

an anxiety disorder who is taking a long-acting drug. In that case, a somewhat higher dose of clorazepate or diazepam may be necessary at bedtime to improve sleep and increase the daytime anxiolytic effect. We do not recommend increasing the dosage of shorter-acting drugs beyond the dosages listed. Rather, if a patient denies that a hypnotic is effective, it is an indication that the treatment is not efficacious and an alternative treatment must be considered. Regardless of the etiology of the insomnia, a reasonable dosage of a benzodiazepine medication should offer some relief. When it does not, two possibilities should be pursued. Insomnia secondary to psychiatric illness often will not respond to a clinical dosage of benzodiazepine medication. Affective illness is the most common psychiatric disorder we see at our sleep disorder center, probably because of the profound effect depression can have on sleep and the patient's perception that his depression is secondary to his or her sleep disorder. Patients with depression often report little or no improvement in sleep symptoms with benzodiazepine treatment. This may also be true of patients with other psychiatric disorders (e.g., borderline personality disorder, chronic schizophrenia).

A second consideration when improvement is denied is that there is a large subjective component to the complaint and the patient is a poor estimator of his sleep time. Some patients may have improved sleep, or even normal sleep, but still continue to report short or disrupted sleep. A sleep recording is needed to address this potential problem.

Another type of initial difficulty is that a patient may quickly regress after an initial improvement. This development may signal a change in the situational stresses that have been contributing to the patient's disturbed sleep. Changes in the patient's psychiatric or medical status might also cause this, and further evaluation should be conducted to rule this out, rather than simply changing medications.

Chronicity. A third factor in determining the duration of action is the number of consecutive nights of administration. Any drug with a half-life over six hours will not be completely eliminated after 24 hours and will build up if used chronically. For this reason, flurazepam does not produce its peak hypnotic effect until the third consecutive night of administration (which makes it a poor choice for intermittent use).

Onset of Effect

Rate of absorption varies among benzodiazepines, and this may also be a factor in drug selection. Rapidly absorbed drugs are helpful when delayed sleep-onset latency is part of the sleep problem, but is not necessary for an insomnia that occurs after sleep onset. In the latter case, drugs that are poorly absorbed, such as oxazepam, may be appropriate, especially for elderly patients who may be at risk for accidents or amnesia with rapid sedation.

Type of Metabolism

Generally, as an individual ages, the duration of action of hypnotics becomes longer (even with dose held constant). Exceptions to this are oxazepam, lorazepam, and temazepam, which have similar elimination curves for both young and old adults (Greenblatt, Shader, Divoll, & Harmatz, 1981). This is because of the simpler metabolic route for these compounds. Oxazepam is slowly absorped, which, together with the simpler metabolism, makes this drug a good choice in the treatment of elderly patients.

Available Dosages

A practical issue that may be relevant for certain patients is the range of dosages available for a specific drug. Some patients may initially require dose adjustment to establish the optimal therapeutic effect with the minimal dosage. More often, dosage is an issue when tapering the medication to discontinue treatment. For example lorazepam, alprazolam, and clorazepate are available in a variety of dosages, but flurazepam, triazolam, and temazepam are available in only two dosages.

METHOD

Once an appropriate drug is selected, it must be used properly by the patient. Besides the pharmacokinetic properties of the drug (as described above), efficacy will also be determined by *how* the medication is taken. The medication should be taken in a way which does not encourage bad sleep hygiene. Our overall goal is to achieve consistency in behavior and sleep. The following guidelines are appropriate for any benzodiazepine that might be selected.

General Rules

1. *Establish a firm, clear regimen.* In our sleep disorder center, we feel that the clinician, not the patient, must decide on the drug and the dosage. Therefore, the patient should not be instructed to "take one or two at bedtime" (even if a low dose is used). This approach gives the patient

permission to make dosage changes, and may lead to escalation of the dose by the patient. A specific treatment plan should be in place and the dosage should be fixed. Changes in dosage may be made based on patient response, but these changes are made by the clinician after consultation with the patient. Escalation of dose by the patient is unacceptable and the patient should be made aware, in advance, that escalation will preclude continuing this treatment. All patients should also be instructed to abstain from alcohol and other central nervous system depressants.

2. *The medication must be taken every night.* This may be our most controversial recommendation. Most patients should use the medication every night during a period of drug treatment, rather than on some arbitrary schedule (e.g., every other night) or on an "as needed" basis. Our goal is to establish a strong pattern of consistently good sleep and thereby strengthen good sleep behavior, as well as diminish negative conditioning. For short-term insomnia (or for short-term administration in a patient with chronic insomnia), a two-to-four-week period of every-night use is more effective at establishing a regular pattern of improved sleep than is intermittent use. Shorter-acting medications can be associated with rebound insomnia on the first night of withdrawal. Therefore, an every-other-night schedule on this type of drug is extremely effective in reinforcing the patient's belief that he is entirely unable to sleep without the benefit of medication. Longer-acting medications may not reach their peak efficacy until the third consecutive night of administration and are therefore most appropriate for chronic use.

The major flaw with as-needed use is that the patient must spend time obsessing about his sleep in the process of deciding whether he needs to take sleeping medication on a given night. This is likely to contribute to the negative conditioning that is seen in psychophysiological insomnia. Clinicians who recommend using hypnotic medication as needed presumably do so because of concerns regarding tolerance. However, several studies have shown continued efficacy with long-term administration of benzodiazepines (Adam, Adamson, Brezinova, Hunter, & Oswald, 1976; Stepanski, Zorick, Kaffeman, Sicklesteel, & Roth, 1982; Oswald, French, Adam, & Gilham, 1982). Patients with mild or episodic insomnia might respond to a "once a week" as-needed schedule, but this will be the exception. In most patients with chronic insomnia, as-needed use will lead to less consistency in sleep and sleep habits.

3. *The medication must be taken 30 minutes before bedtime.* We recommend never having a patient take medication after bedtime. Many times patients first "try to sleep" and take the medication only after lying in bed awake for some time. This is to be avoided because it teaches the patient to lie in bed and obsess about when and if he should arise and take a pill. Instead, the

medication should be taken 15 to 30 minutes before bedtime. If it is not taken before bedtime, then the patient should abstain from using it, even if he is awake all night. For the same reasons, patients should not take repeat dosages during the night. We have seen several patients who only complain of maintenance difficulties and have been instructed to wait until awakening before taking a short-acting medication. This approach guarantees that the patient will awaken every night and stay awake long enough to take medication and wait for it to work. Instead, the patient should take an intermediate-acting drug at bedtime.

4. *Use only one benzodiazepine in a given patient*. There is never a reason to combine different sedative–hypnotic medications or sedative–hypnotic and anxiolytic drugs. It is simpler to manage the patient and to eventually reduce and discontinue the medication if only one drug is used. We see violations of this rule often, usually with psychiatric patients. For example, a patient being treated for an anxiety disorder who also complains of insomnia is given alprazolam, 0.5 mg three times daily, and temazepam 30 mg at bedtime. Instead, he could be given a long-acting drug at bedtime only, or at least multiple doses of the same drug. If it is clinically necessary to prescribe a drug like alprazolam, then the bulk of the daily dosage could be given at bedtime. This would be accomplished in the patient above with alprazolam, 0.5 mg twice daily and 1.0 mg at bedtime. This approach may require that these issues be discussed with another professional who may be treating the psychiatric illness or someone who is prescribing the anxiolytic.

Example Protocols for Specific Diagnoses

These protocols are meant to serve as illustrations of the approach described in this chapter. We again must point out that each patient will have individual characteristics which may require modifications in treatment.

Short-Term Insomnia. When the history of the problem is recent, and the patient previously slept well, then a brief trial of symptomatic treatment with hypnotics may be adequate to return the patient to a regular pattern of good sleep. Start with two weeks of every-night administration of triazolam, 0.125 or 0.25 mg (if sleep onset is the primary problem), or temazepam, 30 mg (if sleep maintenance is poor). Reduce the medication by one-half for the third week and discontinue it by the fourth. This schedule can be more flexible, depending on the situational factors for the specific patient.

Insomnia Secondary to an Anxiety Disorder. Start the patient on clorazepate, 15 mg, or diazepam, 10 mg, 30 minutes before bedtime. If the patient continues to have significant sleep disturbance, the dosage may be increased to clorazepate, 22.5 mg, or diazepam, 15 mg. In patients with severe anxiety disorders, an additional dose during the day may be required. Presumably psychotherapy will also be part of the overall treatment plan, and decisions regarding tapering and discontinuation of the medication should be made in conjunction with the therapist.

Restless Legs/Periodic Leg Movements. Begin treatment with clonazepam, 0.5 mg 30 minutes before bedtime. If, after one week, there is no improvement, the dosage may be increased to 1.0 mg. If, after another week, this is not successful, the dosage should be reduced and the drug finally discontinued. We have not found a patient who did not respond to 1.0 mg who then responded to a higher dosage, although this has been reported by others. Instead, another treatment strategy, such L-dopa, should be considered. If the patient has significant daytime sleepiness, an intermediate-acting drug (e.g., temazepam) may be used initially, instead of clonazepam.

Severe Psychophysiological Insomnia, Childhood-Onset Insomnia, Patients Refractory to Other Treatments. Try lorazepam, 1.0 mg, for one week. This may be increased by 0.5 mg per week increments up to a maximum of 2.0 mg. Lorazepam is suggested because it is effective throughout the sleep period and many dosages are available, but many other benzodiazepines could also be used in this situation.

Insomnia Secondary to Medical Illness, Pain, or Medication. Same as above, except that longer-acting drugs may be more helpful.

Use of Antidepressants

Obviously, if it is determined that a patient's insomnia is secondary to depression, then treatment should be aimed at the affective illness. It is not our intention to provide extensive information regarding the treatment of depression, but because persistent insomnia can frequently be caused by depression we will make some suggestions.

In those patients with depression in whom insomnia is a chief symptom, use of sedating tricyclic antidepressants (TCA) such as amitriptyline or doxepin, is recommended (if there are no medical contraindications). The whole dose (up to 150 mg) can be given one-half to one hour before bedtime, and the side effect of sedation will immediately provide some relief from the insomnia. Many practitioners seem to routinely avoid these drugs in favor of newer antidepressants with fewer side effects. However, patients with severe insomnia complain less of side effects, provided the dose is not increased too quickly. We recommend starting at 50 mg and increasing by 50 mg only after one full week at that dosage.

Then, if clinically indicated, increase by another 50 mg after another full week. We believe that use of these medications is preferable to using a nonsedating TCA. Some clinicians add a benzodiazepine to a nonsedating TCA for symptomatic treatment of insomnia with depression. This is an option if a nonsedating TCA must be used for some reason. Nevertheless, our first choice is treatment with a single medication, in this case a sedating TCA.

For similar reasons, we do not recommend use of the stimulating antidepressants (e.g., protriptyline, fluoxetine, or monoamine oxidase inhibitors) in patients complaining of severe insomnia, unless treatment with other antidepressants has already failed. One must then accept that the insomnia will most likely worsen.

CASE HISTORY

Case 1

Mr. C, a 71-year-old man, 5 feet 6 inches tall and weighing 133 pounds, was referred for insomnia of two years' duration. Prior to that he had slept well. He reported a sleep-onset latency of several hours and an average total sleep time of three to four hours. He complained of discomfort and twitches in his leg muscles prior to sleep onset. Mr. C also reported feeling very sleepy during the day and regularly took a one-to-two hour nap in the afternoon. If he did not nap, he had great difficulty functioning in the afternoon. This patient had a history of chronic hepatitis of unknown etiology with cirrhotic changes in the liver. Alcoholism was denied and this was confirmed by his primary medical doctor (PMD). He also had aseptic necrosis of the left femoral head secondary to chronic use of steroids. His only medications were prednisone, 7.5 mg every day, and Persantine. The patient kept a constant arising time of 8 A.M. and was usually in bed for seven to eight hours. He appeared mildly depressed but psychometric testing [Minnesota Multiphasic Personality Inventory (MMPI)] was unremarkable. Mr. C had been on disability for 15 years because of his medical problems. Despite this, he stayed reasonably active during the day. The patient's wife confirmed that his sleep pattern was as he described.

The patient was told to eliminate his afternoon naps and to stay out of bed at night if unable to sleep (stimulus control suggestions). These changes failed to result in any improvement in the patient's sleep after two weeks of monitoring with sleep logs. He had difficulty skipping his usual nap, but even after he did so for several days, his nighttime sleep did not improve appreciably.

An overnight sleep recording during the patient's usual hours in bed found 4.3 hours of sleep, with many arousals and a high percentage of stage 1 sleep. The arousals either were secondary to periodic leg movements during sleep or were idiopathic. The multiple sleep latency test (MSLT) found moderate to severe daytime sleepiness, with uniformly short latencies to sleep across the day.

The patient was given a trial on oxazepam, 15 mg. This medication was chosen because of the patient's age and liver disease (and the low dosage was used for the same reasons). The concern is that drug accumulation with repeated dosages will occur if drug metabolism is impaired owing to age or liver dysfunction. Oxazepam's duration of action is minimally affected by these variables because of its simpler route of metabolism and excretion.

Mr. C was monitored with sleep logs and twice-weekly phone contact. The logs showed improved sleep, with an average total sleep time of seven hours. After one week, he also reported feeling more alert during the day and was able to stop taking naps. After one month, the medication was discontinued. The patient continued to complete logs and slept well for one week, but then his poor sleep returned. Two weeks later he was restarted on oxazepam, 15 mg. He took the medication every night for four months with consistently good sleep and was referred back to his PMD for ongoing care.

Case 2

In another example, a 32-year-old man was referred for insomnia of about 20 years' duration. He stated that he sometimes had a long sleep onset latency, but more often had frequent awakenings during the night and often had difficulty returning to sleep. At times he also awakened too early and was unable to return to sleep. He complained of daytime tiredness and difficulty concentrating. He denied use of alcohol and denied napping. This patient drank three cups of coffee each morning. He went to bed at 9:30 P.M. and arouse at 4:30 A.M. because he could not get any more sleep, even though he did not have to be up to get ready for work until 5:30 A.M. He had used triazolam, 0.25 mg, in the past, which he felt improved his sleep, but he still did not feel his best during the day. He denied feeling depressed and stated that his appetite was good and his weight was stable. However, he reported that he has always been "hyper" and likes to be "on the go."

The patient appeared jittery and anxious, but denied any cognitive symptoms of anxiety. His only medical problem was chronic bronchitis, which he felt was caused by his poor sleep. He had been treated previously with relaxation training and behavioral monitoring. He believed that this allowed him to relax better in bed, but he did not sleep any longer or deeper. He was not articulate, lacked psychological insight, and was not judged to be a good candidate for traditional psychotherapy. In fact, he had seen a therapist once in the past and felt he had not benefitted.

On a sleep recording, the patient slept 3.5 hours, with a high percentage of light sleep. He had many idiopathic arousals and awakenings distributed across the night. A long-acting hypnotic, flurazepam, 30 mg, was prescribed. This drug was used because the patient appeared somewhat anxious during the day and would therefore benefit from the mild daytime sedation that accompanies use of flurazepam, 30 mg. The patient reported improved sleep for several months. This improvement was confirmed by polysomnography, which found a total sleep time of six hours with much less light sleep and fewer awakenings. Upon discontinuation of the medication, the patient reported worsened sleep after three nights, which would be consistent with the slow decline in blood level after chronic use that is characteristic of this drug. When his sleep had not improved at all after two weeks the medication was restarted.

The patient has now taken flurazepam, 30 mg, for 2.5 years with continued efficacy. At one point, about one year after initiation of treatment, the patient reported that he was not sleeping as well as he originally did after starting the medication. He was again asked to keep sleep logs, and they revealed that the patient had changed his work hours. His sleep schedule now required him to go to bed three hours earlier than before and he was returning to his old schedule on weekends. He was put on a regular sleep–wake schedule and after about ten days was sleeping well again. Once per year, the medication has been withdrawn for two weeks, and each time his sleep has become short and fragmented by multiple awakenings.

DISCUSSION

Drug Discontinuation

We recommend gradual tapering of the drug to avoid withdrawal effects, such as rebound insomnia, which is a worsening of sleep beyond even baseline levels upon drug withdrawal. This effect is more likely to occur with shorter-acting drugs and following use of larger doses. Rebound insomnia has been found even after only one night of administration. Tapering of the dose is less likely to cause withdrawal effects than is abrupt discontinuation. For example, for a patient taking triazolam, 0.25 mg, we would reduce the dosage to 0.125 mg for a full week before discontinuing the drug altogether.

Contraindications

Certain patients are not candidates for treatment with hypnotics, despite the failure of other approaches or other apparent indications. Presence of the following conditions should be carefully explored before treatment.

Definitely exclude from drug treatment:
1. History of alcoholism or drug abuse
2. History of benzodiazepine abuse
3. History of an adverse reaction to benzodiazepines

May have adverse effects:
1. Certain psychiatric disorders, especially borderline personality disorder, schizophrenia, or other psychoses
2. Pulmonary disease, which may be worsened by sedation
3. Liver disease, which may change drug metabolism

Side Effects

The incidence of side effects increases with the size of the dose. Even at therapeutic dosages, however, some patients may have side effects such as blurred vision, dizziness, morning grogginess, memory impairment, or slurred speech. Reducing the dosage may be helpful; if the effect is severe, drug discontinuation is recommended.

SUMMARY

Hypnotic efficacy in the treatment of many causes of insomnia has been established for benzodiazepine medication. However, tolerance may develop with chronic administration (longer than four weeks), and the benefits must be weighed against potential side effects, including memory impairment, daytime sedation, and morning "hangover." In those cases where hypnotics are to be used, care should be given to select the proper drug and dosage to suit the individual patient and type of sleep problem. These drugs vary in duration of effect, onset of effect, and type of metabolism. Success of treatment will also rely on giving the patient proper instructions regarding use of the medication. Any escalation of dosage by the patient is unacceptable and should result in consideration of other treatment alternatives.

Edward J. Stepanski earned a Ph.D. in clinical psychology from Bowling Green State University in 1985, since which time he has been Director of the Insomnia Clinic at the Henry Ford Hospital (HFH) Sleep Disorders and Research Center. The HFH Sleep center was established in 1978 and now evaluates approximately 1400 new patients each year.

Frank J. Zorick is a Board-Certified psychiatrist and the Medical Director of HFH Sleep Disorder and Research Center. Dr. Zorick has been evaluating patients with sleep complaints on a full-time basis since 1978.

Thomas Roth is Founder and Director of the HFH Sleep Disorder and Research Center and a past President of the American Sleep Disorders Association. He is a psychologist and has published over 80 articles in the area of pharmacology and sleep.

RECOMMENDED READINGS

Greenblatt, D. J., Shader, R. I., Divoll, M., & Harmatz, J. S. (1981). Benzodiazepines: A summary of pharmokinetic properties. *British Journal of Clinical Pharmacology, 11,* 11S–16S.
  This paper describes the pharmokinetics of various benzodiazepine medications. Special emphasis is given to single-dose effects as opposed to multiple-dose effects, and the specific differences between drugs are discussed.
Nicholson, A. N. (1989). Hypnotics: Clinical pharmacology and therapeutics. In M. H. Kryger, T. Roth, & W. C. Dement (Eds.), *Principles and practice of sleep medicine*. Philadelphia: W. B. Saunders, pp. 219–228.
  This chapter provides a description of the relevant pharmacology of hypnotic drugs. It also provides detailed summaries of the individual differences between various hypnotic medications. Finally, there are recommendations on the appropriate clinical use of these drugs.
Woods, J. H., Katz, J. L., & Winger, G. (1988). Use and abuse of benzodiazepines: Issues relevant to prescribing. *Journal of the American Medical Association, 260*(23), 3476–3480.
  This paper reviews the literature in regard to potential dependence with benzodiazepine use. Adverse effects are also discussed.

REFERENCES

Adam, K., Adamson, L., Brezinova, V., Hunter, W., & Oswald, I. (1976). Nitrazepam: Lastingly effective but trouble on withdrawal. *British Medical Journal, 1,* 1558–1560.

Bornstein, P., & Cujo, P. (1974). Influence of barbiturates and benzodiazepines on the sleep EEG. In T. M. Itil, (Ed.), *Psychotropic drugs and the human EEG. Modern problems of pharmacopsychiatry (Vol. 8)*. Basel: Karger, pp. 182–192.

Greenblatt, D. J. (1980). Pharmacokinetic comparisons. *Psychosomatics, 21*(10), 9–14.

Greenblatt, D., Shader, R., Divoll, M., & Harmatz, J. (1981). Benzodiazepines: A summary of pharmacokinetic properties. *British Journal of Clinical Pharmacology, 11*, 11S–16S.

Johnson, L. C., & Chernik, D. A. (1982). Sedative–hypnotics and human performance. *Psychopharmacology, 76*, 101–114.

Kales, A., Kales, J. D., Bixler, E. O., & Scharf, M. B. (1975). Effectiveness of hypnotic drugs with prolonged use: Flurazepam and pentobarbital. *Clinical Pharmacology and Therapeutics, 18*, 356–363.

Moskowitz, H., & Smiley, A. (1982). Effects of chronically administered buspirone and diazepam on driving-related skills performance. *Journal of Clinical Psychiatry, 43*(12), 45–55.

National Institute of Mental Health, Consensus Development Conference. (1984). Drugs and insomnia: The use of medications to promote sleep. *Journal of the American Medical Association, 251*, 2410–2414.

Nicholson, A. N. (1981). The use of short- and long-acting hypnotics in clinical medicine. *British Journal of Clinical Pharmacology, 11*, 61S–69S.

Oswald, I., French, C., Adam, K., & Gilham, J. (1982). Benzodiazepine hypnotics remain effective for 24 weeks. *British Medical Journal, 284*, 860–863.

Perkins, R., & Hinton, J. (1974). Sedative or tranquilizer? A comparison of the hypnotic effects of chlordiazepoxide and amylobarbitone sodium. *British Journal of Psychiatry, 124*, 435–439.

Roehrs, T., Kribbs, N., Zorick, F., & Roth, T. (1986). Hypnotic residual effects of benzodiazepines with repeated administration. *Sleep, 9*(2), 309–316.

Roehrs, T., Vogel, G., Wittig, R., Zorick, F., Paxton, C., Lamphere, J., & Roth, T. (1986). Dose effects of temazepam tablets on sleep. *Drugs in Experimental Clinical Research, 12*(8), 693–699.

Roehrs, T., Zorick, F., Sicklesteel, J., Wittig, R., Hartse, K., & Roth, T. (1983). Effects of hypnotics on memory. *Journal of Clinical Pharmacology, 3*(5), 310–313.

Roth, T., Hartse, K. M., Saab, P. G., Piccione, P. M., & Kramer, M. (1980). The effects of flurazepam, lorazepam, and triazolam on sleep and memory. *Psychopharmacology, 70*, 231–237.

Stepanski, E., Zorick, F., Kaffeman, M., Sicklesteel, J., & Roth, T. (1982). Effects of the chronic administration of triazolam 0.50 mg on the sleep of insomniacs. *Nouvelle Presse Médicale, 11*, 2987–2990.

Veldkamp, W., Straw, R. N., Metzler, C. M., & Demissianos, H. V. (1974). Efficacy and residual effect evaluation of a new hypnotic, triazolam. *Journal of Clinical Pharmacology, 14*, 102–111.

Vogel, G. W., Barker, K., Gibbons, P., & Thurmond, A. (1976). A comparison of the effects of flurazepam 30 mgs and triazolam 0.5 mgs on the sleep of insomniacs. *Psychopharmacologia, 47*, 81–86.

Part Three

Comprehensive and Integrated Approaches

Parts One and Two deal with individual treatment methods for insomnia. However, we have emphasized all along that no competent insomnia therapist will restrict him/herself to one or the other technique alone. Rather, elements of different techniques are typically combined in the overall treatment strategy, depending on the needs of the patient and depending on the therapist's background and experience. Chapters Nine through Eleven summarize three ways in which this can be done.

Stevenson and Weinstein's chapter emphasizes that such a program has to originate from the patient's perceptive and has to be individualized to meet the patient's specific needs. Therefore, assessment is stressed and an effort is made to help the patients conceptualize their sleep problem in a new way. Education is a main goal, and a "model of a good night's sleep" is presented. Various treatment approaches are used, depending on the patient's needs, and no two patients get the same treatment. Stevenson and Weinstein stress that it is important to help patients succeed where they have previously failed and to initially emphasize even minimal progress.

In Chapter Ten, Steinberg emphasizes the importance of the vicious cycle in insomnia: emotional stress leading to physiological arousal, which results in sleeplessness and increased emotional stress. The individual emotional reaction to sleep loss directs at least part of the treatment, and maladaptive coping styles are frequently the focus of psychotherapeutic approaches in these individuals.

Nau, Koewler, and Walsh discuss sleep behavior management in Chapter Eleven. They attempt to identify behavioral changes that would be likely to improve sleep. They then implement these changes, using behavioral therapy principles in the context of a therapeutic alliance with the patient. Knowledge and education are stressed not only to help patients overcome the current problem, but also to fortify them for future sleep disturbances and to help them feel less helpless.

CHAPTER NINE

Selecting a Treatment Strategy

MICHAEL M. STEVENSON AND MARSHA K. WEINSTEIN

INTRODUCTION

Patients complaining of insomnia are a fairly heterogeneous group, with multiple factors causing and maintaining their sleeplessness. We find it helpful in selecting an optimal treatment strategy to understand insomnia from the patient's perspective. Understanding how insomnia has been conceptualized, what coping strategies have been selected, and the role it has come to play in the patient's life provides useful information as to how insomnia can best be treated. The patient's own selection of a coping strategy is often determined by how the insomnia is perceived and evaluated. This is partly a function of the patient's belief system about his or her ability to sleep and to function without sleep.

Some patients may report multiple factors causing their sleep difficulty. They may experience several stressors (e.g., loss of job, illness, death of a family member, time zone change, etc.) before any chronic insomnia problem emerges. Some may report a single stressor that periodically repeats itself (final exams, vacations, workshift change, etc.) making insomnia worse with each occurrence. In other patients chronic insomnia may develop much more slowly and have no clear precipitating event. The patient may report only a vague, amorphous loss of sleeping ability over a long period of time lasting several months to years.

In our experience, whether or not patients convert from transient to

---

Michael M. Stevenson and Marsha K. Weinstein • North Valley Sleep Disorders Center, Mission Hills, California 91345.

chronic insomnia depends on their conceptualization of their sleep problem, personality, and previous sleep experience. Patients who conceptualize their insomnia with beliefs like "I can't function without sleep" or "When I don't sleep people will notice how awful I look" are more likely to develop a chronic sleeping difficulty than patients who have attached less importance to their sleep. When sleep does not meet their expectations, they view themselves as having failed. Negative self-statements lead to the negative emotions of frustration, irritability, anger, and anxiety, with an associated arousal of the nervous system and an inability to sleep. Patients who are poor at problem solving or who feel a helpless loss of control may be more likely to see insomnia as an unsolvable problem. An underlying psychiatric disturbance, such as an anxiety or affective or personality disorder, indicates the presence of limited coping resources to deal with insomnia. Prior negative "sleep experiences" or what family members or friends say about their own sleep experience also contribute to a sense of feeling isolated and helpless in solving the insomnia problem.

Patients have frequently tried various coping strategies by the time they have reached our office. Some of these were self-generated, others were suggestions by friends or family members, others by articles in books or magazines, and still others by previous professional contacts (physicians, mental health professionals, hypnotherapists, etc.). Many patients have actually tried various widely recognized standard treatments with limited success. Some have been in psychotherapy for months to years with no change in their sleep. Patient-coping strategies typically fall into two categories: behavioral and drug. Behavioral strategies include common methods, such as reading and watching television until sleepy, spending extra time in bed either by going to bed early or by sleeping late, taking warm baths, listening to relaxation tapes, meditating, and using distracting images. Some patients have self-medicated with alcohol or over-the-counter sleep preparations or are currently habituated to a prescription sleeping pill.

We believe that the main reason patients fail at solving their insomnia problem is lack of a clear understanding of the phenomenon of sleep and what's needed for a good night's sleep. Some patients try various widely recognized techniques to control insomnia, such as stimulus control or relaxation exercises (Bootzin & Nicassio, 1978), but fail for one reason or another. They may be inconsistent, may give up too soon, or may be treating only part of their problem. We provide patients with our model of a good night's sleep and then explore with them what's lacking in their sleep behavior as well as which coping strategies are needed to set the appropriate conditions for sleep to occur. Our model of a good night's sleep identifies five attributes needed to sleep well on a regular basis:

1. A positive association between one's bedroom and sleep
2. An ability to relax
3. A regular sleep/wake circadian rhythm
4. Sleepiness at bedtime
5. Minimal internal and external disturbances to sleep

Patients are given various exercises to improve their sleep which take into account the attributes missing from our good sleep model. Standard exercises are often modified to account for a patient's age, personality, style of coping, and secondary symptoms. Treatment generally takes four to eight weeks.

ASSESSMENT

As there are many causes and contributing factors to the maintenance of chronic insomnia, it is important to perform a thorough assessment. This is not only necessary for purposes of differential diagnosis (ruling out other psychiatric disorders, medical problems, or other sleep disorders), but it is essential for the development of a successful treatment strategy. Insomnia is best treated from a multidimensional approach that is specific to a patient's individual personality, style of coping, age, sleep experiences, secondary symptoms, and deviation from the model of a good sleeper. Although assessment can be seen as an ongoing process, we attempt to obtain as much background information as possible in the first session. Patients complete a sleep/wake questionnaire to aid in this process.

How patients conceptualize their sleep, the impact it has had on their life, and what they expect from treatment serve as a starting point in the assessment process. Patients are asked to describe their sleep problem and how they would like it changed. How the problem is stated gives us an idea of how realistic patients may be in their expectations of treatment and indicates any preconceived notions they may have about sleep. Statements such as "I want to sleep eight hours per night and not wake up" may be unrealistic, depending on the age of the patient.

Asking patients to list the daytime symptoms they experience will also give the therapist an idea of what treatments might be most effective. Some report no daytime symptoms at all, in spite of claiming to sleep very little at night. These patients may actually misperceive how much they sleep or actually need substantially less sleep than average to function normally. Others may report severe difficulties in concentrating on even the simplest of tasks following a poor night's sleep. Poor sleepers are more likely than normal sleepers to misperceive their conscious states and therefore tend to overestimate their sleep onset time as well as underestimate their total sleep time (Carskadon, Dement, Mittler, Guilleminault, Zarcone, & Spiegel, 1976).

We also assess how the patients' friends and family react to their problem and how they sleep in comparison. This is especially important when dealing with a married patient, whose spouse is often someone who falls asleep quickly and doesn't awaken until morning. Having a knowledge of the patient's sleep frame of reference also helps in selecting what educational information needs to be conveyed.

A detailed history of the patient's sleep problem should be obtained, including when the insomnia started, the precipitating event(s), and the symptom intensity. Often, some stressful life event, such as a death, illness, separation, or move to a new residence, can be identified. Sometimes a cumulative series of events creates enough stress to cause the sleep problem. Patients, especially those who have had insomnia for many years, may have difficulty remembering a single precipitating event. Memories can be jogged by asking what major life changes may have occurred when insomnia began. Identifying stressors can be helpful later when patients learn how to recognize their stress level and to self-manage future difficulties with sleep. Questions about how the insomnia has fit into their life and the effect it has had on decision making and on personal relationships help us understand the impact of this disorder over a span of many years.

We question the patients in detail about their sleep habits, what time they go to bed, their sleep-onset time, if they wake up and for how long, what they do when they wake up, what time they wake up, and what time they get out of bed in the morning. Asking about the variability of the sleep schedule is always important. Does the patient sleep late some days, go to bed at different hours, or take naps? Having patients specify what happens as they attempt to go to sleep, when and how they know they're sleepy, and what wakes them up at night can give clues as to what treatment strategy will be most effective. For example, patients may report feeling sleepy and unable to focus attention while watching television in the living room but suddenly feel "wired" and unable to sleep only minutes later in the bedroom, demonstrating a negative association between the bedroom and the act of sleeping. Important treatment information may also be obtained by paying close attention to how patients organize their presleep activities. Some patients may allow very little transition time between the activities of the day and any attempt to sleep. Others may spend the entire evening carefully planning their sleep, with any unexpected deviation from their rituals resulting in insomnia.

We identify medical problems, their impact on a patient's life, and how they may be contributing to insomnia. For example, chronic pain related to a number of physical problems, such as arthritis, poor circulation, back problems, or headaches, may produce sleeplessness. In older patients, medical problems and the drugs used to treat them often play a large role in the disruption of sleep. Sleep may also be affected by worry about health. Sometimes, the beginnings of insomnia can be traced to surgery or illness that dramatically changed the patient's activity level, caused a great deal of anxiety, or involved a postoperative trial of sleeping medication.

The patient's present and past dependence on any sleeping medication is thoroughly assessed. The patient fills out a questionnaire outlining the use of caffeine, alcohol, and tobacco. All these substances have been found to affect sleep (Curatolo & Robertson, 1983; Soldatos, Kales, Scharf, Bixler, & Kales, 1980; Zarcone, 1989). We assess the use of prescription drugs and over-the-counter medications for impact on the patient's sleep.

Insomnia is a major diagnostic characteristic for a number of psychiatric disorders (American Psychiatric Association, 1987). It is therefore important to have detailed knowledge about any associated psychiatric disturbances. Patients with insomnia sometimes display tearfulness or sadness and voice complaints of feeling angry and depressed. In a patient who is not experiencing a major depression, these symptoms will usually lift within a few weeks of treatment. The clinically depressed patient tends not to respond to our treatment program alone and requires referral for consideration of antidepressant medication.

Symptoms of insomnia may be produced by sleep apnea, nocturnal myoclonus, or restless legs (American Sleep Disorders Association Diagnostic Classification Steering Committee, 1990). A number of questions are asked of the patient to rule out these disorders. In addition, a questionnaire is filled out by the bed partner to find out if any unusual behaviors have been noticed. We are looking for symptoms such as periodic leg movements or behaviors such as snoring, pauses in breathing, or snorting noises which indicate possible sleep apnea. If it is suspected that one of these or other sleep disorders may be present, a nocturnal polysomnogram is recommended.

Patients with insomnia vary widely in their sleep habits and their reaction to not sleeping well. They all, however, attempt some kind of adjustments to their sleep problem, usually without success. Information is gathered on what coping strategies patients have tried and the subsequent impact on their sleep. For example, some patients get into bed early because they are so tired, but this only serves to lengthen their sleep-onset time. To know how many times a particular technique was tried before it was discarded will be helpful in determining its usefulness in future treatment. We assess the patient's level of frustration in reaction to coping failures. Some patients are quite objective and methodical in their approach to solutions. Others are more impulsive and emotional. Their coping style gives us a clue as to how much intervention a patient may tolerate, how slowly treatment should proceed, and the emotional support needed for success.

The life-style or the general psychosocial atmosphere in which the individual lives and works has a profound impact on the treatment process. It includes the pace, stress level, and relaxation opportunities in one's everyday life. We look at family structure (married, unmarried, children), work environment, and social contacts. We look for opportunities for support and comfort. We attempt to find out the amount of stress experienced, its sources, and how it is handled. We focus on opportunities for relaxation, socializing, private time, and exercise. Sensitivity to personal life-style differences can help the therapist avoid treatment methods and approaches that prove too difficult for the patient to accommodate and set the pace of treatment at a level that will ensure maximum compliance.

In the initial phase of treatment, the therapist is often dealing with the emotional fallout of chronic insomnia. The patient is depressed and anxious and feels an overwhelming loss of control. Although patients will exhibit a wide range of emotional reactions in response to their insomnia, some anxiety about their poor sleep is nearly universal. This anxiety can often be the greatest barrier to producing better sleep. If therapists can pinpoint the source of a patient's anxiety, they can help him/her learn to deal with it more effectively. For instance, if you ask a patient, "What is the worst thing that will happen if you don't sleep?" you may elicit a response such as, "I won't be able to function at work." With further questioning, you may find that the patient is able to perform work tasks, but does not feel very energetic or sharp. Patients may worry that others will notice that they are sleepy or think they are acting strangely. They then may avoid others or take on fewer responsibilities. If anxiety about the detrimental effects of a loss of sleep can be addressed and reduced, some of the anxiety about insomnia will lessen. With the subsequent reduction of pressure to sleep well, a patient is more likely to be able to relax and fall asleep.

We attempt to assess what issues may be operating to prevent change. Although patients may seem motivated, they may be unwilling to give up insomnia because of "secondary gain." For example, in some patients, the only time they can work out problems is in the middle of the night, when family members are asleep. Sometimes insomnia can prevent an individual from making a career move or starting a new relationship because of anticipatory anxiety. It can become a roadblock that prevents individuals from taking on certain responsibilities. For example, being continuously late for work because of sleeping late can be a way of passively expressing anger about certain job or school dissatisfactions.

A patient's personality, emotional coping skills, anxiety level, and motivation are all factors that have an impact on the approach and pace of treatment. With highly anxious, emotionally upset patients, more time giving reassurance and emotional support is needed. For some individuals used to solving problems from a practical viewpoint, treatment may be more goal-oriented and behavioral. It is important to give patients a feeling of success where they have previously failed, thereby reinforcing their attempts to change. It also means that assessment is an ongoing process, with the flexibility to change treatment in response to patient needs. There can be a delicate balance between encouraging a patient to continue an intervention that may be uncomfortable in the hope of providing future success versus knowing when to abandon an approach as too stressful.

TREATMENT

In our treatment program we help the patient develop a constructive, positive conceptualization of his/her sleep, as well as promote the development of sleep-enhancing coping strategies. The patient is more likely to be able to accomplish this if the following criteria are met: First, the patient is educated about normal sleep: what it is, what enhances it, what prevents it. Second, both the patient and therapist understand why the patient's insomnia developed and what has maintained it. Third, our model of a good night's sleep becomes integrated into the patient's conceptualization of sleep. Knowledge about sleep, combined with an understanding of why coping strategies fail and how they can be corrected, gives patients a sense of control. This helps them regain confidence and reduces anxiety even following a poor night's sleep. Use of treatment techniques that support our model of a good night's sleep leads to the development of new coping strategies and improved sleep.

Education about Normal Sleep

Most patients have little knowledge about sleep or the prevalence of sleeping problems in the general population. Patients experiencing chronic insomnia often feel isolated and "sick." Their view of their insomnia as a disease results in increased anxiety. The information provided to patients is aimed at helping them reduce their anxiety about sleep by understanding it better. Many patients "try too hard to go to sleep." We emphasize the concept that sleep is an involuntary process and that the harder they try to sleep, the more likely they will fail. We stress that the patient cannot "control" sleep directly, but can only set the ideal conditions for it to occur.

We address the perception of waking versus sleep. Some people who experience insomnia may actually be unaware that they are asleep. Other patients are concerned why awakenings occur at certain times of the night. We explain about sleep architecture and the various stages of sleep. We also explain about their biological clock and sleep, as well as the synchronization of their circadian rhythm with light and various sociopsychological cues (Dinges, 1989).

Some patients are concerned about the harmful effects of sleep deprivation. They are often fearful that they will become ill or may be causing great physical harm. We relate to patients that no evidence exists for any serious long-lasting effects from loss of sleep (Horne, 1988).

Many patients seen at the Sleep Disorders Center are still expecting themselves to sleep as long and as deeply as when they were children. We explain how sleep changes over time, emphasizing the decline in sleep efficiency with age. We also explain that an individual's sleep will become lighter and more fragmented as he or she grows older (Reynolds, Kupfer, Taska, Hock, Sewitch, & Spiker, 1985). This is especially important when dealing with the elderly, but is relevant for all individuals over 40.

Patients are also educated about the effects of alcohol and tobacco on sleep. We also discuss the impact of long-term use of sleeping pills in decreasing the patient's ability to fall asleep naturally. With increased use, drug tolerance may develop and the dosage must be increased to produce the same results (Nicholson, 1989). This can result in more daytime fatigue and/or sleepiness. Individuals also have increased difficulty falling asleep naturally as they become more drug dependent. If they try to stop taking these medications, they experience "rebound insomnia" and become more convinced that they can't sleep without pills.

Learning about Their Own Insomnia

Each week patients fill out a detailed record of their sleep on a sleep diary. On this record, they write down bedtime, sleep-onset time, number of times awakened, amount of time awake during the night, final waking time, total hours slept, and sleep quality. There is a "comments" section for the patient to note any stressors during the day or other factors that may have an effect on their sleep (going out late at night, fight with spouse, etc.). The sleep diary provides both the therapist and the patient with a concrete record of sleep during treatment and serves as the basis for treatment modifications. Patients report that it is helpful to refer back to a previous record in which they experienced poor sleep and were able to recover and sleep well the next night. The comments section is particularly useful in helping the patients identify specific events or issues that lead to poor sleep.

Model of a Good Night's Sleep

Patients learn that certain factors set the state for sleep to occur, and instead of using energy to try to make themselves sleep, they focus on "letting sleep happen." This becomes an important change in a patient's viewpoint. Patients learn to focus on areas over which there is control, i.e., the factors that enhance the possibility for sleep to occur. The five areas of focus in the model of a good night's sleep provide the basis for "setting the stage" for sleep.

Positive Association between Bedroom and Act of Sleeping. The most common deviation from the model of a good night's sleep in a poor sleeper is the negative association between the bedroom and the act of sleeping. This has developed and been strengthened over a period of time. By the time patients are seen in treatment, they view their bedroom as a "torture chamber" where they spend hours as prisoners, tossing and turning throughout the night. If a patient reports that "the minute I get into bed I am wide awake," you know you are dealing with a negative association with the bedroom. Before success can occur, this conditioned association must be changed from a negative to a positive one.

1. **Stimulus control**: We use stimulus control (Bootzin & Nicassio, 1978) as one of our techniques to correct this problem, but often modify the standard instructions to increase compliance. If not sleepy, we suggest that patients stay up later than usual to ensure that they are actually "ready" for sleep. If they have not fallen asleep within 10 to 30 minutes, we suggest they get up and relax out of the bedroom until sleepy, but for no more than 30 minutes, and then return to bed again. In our experience this lessens the chance of patients falling asleep out of the bedroom, increases compliance, and works more quickly by increasing the number of "learning trials." What patients do to relax is individualized (i.e., reading, listening to music, watching television).

2. **Sleep restriction**: Some patients attempt to "make up" for lost sleep by spending more time in bed. This only increases their insomnia. These patients are told instead to "restrict" their time in bed. We provide the standard instructions (Spielman, Saskin, & Thorpy, 1987), but modify them for most patients to obtain more compliance. We find that just limiting time in bed by one or two hours at bedtime will shorten sleep latency and increase sleep efficiency. Sleep restriction often works better than stimulus control with very anxious patients.

3. **Creation of sleep rituals**: The act of getting into bed and going to sleep can be strengthened through the repetition of existing sleep rituals or the creation of new ones. Sleep rituals can provide a behavioral transition that is positive, familiar, and reassuring. It signals to us that we are setting the stage for sleep to occur. We discuss the patients' sleep rituals in some

detail to help them be cognizant of their thoughts and behaviors. Rituals can include specific behaviors, such as teeth brushing, reading, or arranging the bed. Specific thoughts or images regularly repeated at bedtime become associated with falling asleep. In individuals who fall asleep quickly but later experience sleep maintenance difficulties, we have them recreate their original bedtime rituals facilitating the return to sleep. We help them add new ones if there seems to be poverty of rituals in their bedtime routine.

Ability to Relax and Reduce Physiological and Cognitive Arousal States. We address extensively the impact of arousal states on producing and maintaining insomnia. The patient is taught that in order to sleep one must be relaxed both physically and cognitively. Which techniques are used depends on the nature of the patient's state of arousal. Some of the techniques are geared to cognitive processes, others to physiological relaxation.

1. **Physical exercise**: We encourage inactive patients to become involved in some form of aerobic exercise. We start with their current level of physical activity and work up to 30 to 45 minutes four to five times per week. Again, this must be modified depending on the age and physical condition of the patients. Often walking is the easiest and least demanding form of aerobic activity. A late-afternoon or early-evening activity seems to have the most positive effect on sleep (Horne & Porter, 1976).

2. **Deep breathing**: We teach deep breathing (Smith, 1985) as one of the first steps in learning to relax at bedtime. When patients get into bed at night, we ask them to practice slow, even, relaxed diaphragmatic breathing. We often suggest an image to be visualized along with breathing, such as a balloon inflating and deflating. This exercise helps the tense patient achieve a more relaxed physiological state, provides a distraction from intruding thoughts, and helps prevent the occurrence of anxiety symptoms. Many patients like this exercise as it is simple to master and provides immediate results.

3. **Progressive muscle relaxation**: Tense or anxious patients are given an audiotape to teach relaxation. The tape uses a combination of progressive muscle relaxation (Jacobson, 1974) and guided imagery.

4. **Time management**: Some patients are highly stressed because they expect themselves to be able to accomplish too many tasks in a day. We help patients to be realistic in their expectations and learn to define more achievable goals by establishing priorities, setting limits, and developing a realistic time management schedule (McMullen, 1986).

5. **Cognitive restructuring**: Some patients are stressed as a result of irrational or faulty thinking about their sleep. Cognitive restructuring shifts the patients' perceptions from those that are unrealistic and negative to those that are rational and positive. This reduces stress and produces emotional states more conducive to sleep. Many cognitive restructuring

techniques are available to help patients overcome insomnia (Mahoney, 1974). We most often use countering techniques which have the patients argue repeatedly against their irrational thoughts about their sleep until they become weaker, replacing them with positive thoughts.

6. **Problem diary**: For patients who cannot identify stressors in their life ("nothing bothers me") or for those who feel overwhelmed by problems, we recommend that they complete a "problem diary." This exercise consists of taking five to ten minutes in the early evening to write down any problems or concerns, with possible solutions. They may also note a time the next day to further think about the problem. If they awaken during the night and experience "mind racing," the same procedure is carried out. This helps the patient identify concerns *prior* to bedtime, and the act of writing the thoughts down tends, with practice, to remove them from the bedroom.

7. **Thought stopping**: Many patients report that their greatest difficulty in going to sleep is preventing the intrusion of thoughts. These patients complain, "I can't get my mind to stop." Sometimes these thoughts are emotionally charged issues that cause the patient much concern. Other times, they may be fairly benign, such as what chores need to be accomplished the next day. Thought stopping teaches these patients how to "get rid of" unwanted thoughts on command (Mahoney, 1974). The patients practice thinking of unwanted thoughts and, after a short time, clear their mind, using the commands "stop" or "no" to interrupt the negative thoughts. Once thought stopping is learned, thought substitution can be used to replace negative thoughts with pleasant, relaxing images. The purpose of the exercise is to teach patients experiencing obsessive thinking that although they cannot directly control sleep, they can control their thoughts. Learning to be able to stop thinking about something stimulating and replacing those thoughts with images that are relaxing is crucial to reducing cognitive arousal.

8. **Reduction of Stimulation before bedtime**: In order to achieve an optimal state of relaxation at bedtime, a transition period from the day's activities should be instituted. For those patients who do not allow enough relaxation prior to bed, we recommend at least one hour of quiet activity prior to bedtime. For individuals particularly sensitive to stimulation, we suggest avoidance of certain high-arousal (either because of noise level or impact of subject matter) television shows late in the evening. We discuss changes in their evening schedule that will reduce their level of stimulation and maximize relaxation. We sometimes discover that there are late phone calls, arguments with a spouse, work brought home, or involvement in a stimulating hobby prior to bed. For example, one patient worked on his model airplanes late into the night. Setting a time limit on the activity and providing one hour of reading prior to bed improved his sleep dramatically.

Regular Sleep–Wake Circadian Rhythm. Some patients display irregular sleep–wake patterns or patterns out of synch with their ideal sleep period. A common habit is to go to bed when tired but before one is actually sleepy. Patients then lie in bed for hours before falling asleep. Other individuals regularly go to bed too late, not allowing themselves enough time to sleep prior to their scheduled rising time. This puts pressure on them to fall asleep quickly and results in physiological arousal with subsequent sleep-onset problems. These patients frequently sleep late on the weekends to make up for lost sleep during the week. This moves their biological clock forward, reduces their sleepiness, and results in severe insomnia on Sunday night. For patients whose bedtime has been advanced several hours forward from the desired time, we recommend chronotherapy (Czeisler, Richardson, Coleman, Zimmerman, Moore-Ede, Dement, & Weitzman, 1981). In this technique bedtimes are delayed by two- to four-hour increments each night until the desired bedtime is reached. We emphasize that patients should get out of bed in the morning within 30 minutes of the same time each day no matter how little they have slept. We ask patients to avoid sleeping late on weekends in order to regularize their circadian rhythm. We place less emphasis on their bedtime and tell patients that a range of up to two hours is acceptable. They are to find an optimal time when they fall asleep the fastest yet obtain enough sleep to feel good the next day.

Sleepiness at Bedtime. Patients vary as to their awareness of their own sleepiness. At one extreme are those who claim they never feel sleepy. They always feel tired, but no matter when they attempt to sleep, they can't. They also claim they never fall asleep accidentally while watching television, reading, driving, or at a movie. These patients often benefit from keeping a Stanford Sleepiness Scale Diary (Hoddes, Zarcone, Smythe, Phillips, & Dement, 1973), in which they evaluate their alertness on a seven-point scale every hour throughout their waking hours. They learn to pay closer attention to their conscious states and to correlate cognitive and emotional states with environmental conditions. Some of these patients may also be short sleepers and are going to bed before they're actually sleepy. Others may not have an insomnia problem at all, but another medical condition producing symptoms of fatigue during the day. In patients who report no symptoms of fatigue or sleepiness but just an inability to sleep, an all-night sleep recording may reveal that they are sleeping much more than they think.

Minimizing Internal and External Disturbances to Sleep. During the assessment phase the therapist should set as a major goal the discovery of any internal processes (physiological symptoms, medical conditions, sleep disorders, drugs, etc.) which may be disturbing to a patient's sleep.

SELECTING A TREATMENT STRATEGY

The treatment and subsequent reduction or elimination of these factors will aid sleep enormously. For example, helping older patients deal with pain and discomfort during their sleep period will frequently increase sleep efficiency. Many patients try to sleep in environmental conditions not ideally suited to sound sleep. Patients may have spouses who keep them awake by snoring. Helping the patients deal with sleeping in a separate bedroom or getting treatment for the spouses will decrease their insomnia. The reduction of noise through earplugs and white-noise generators is often helpful.

SUCCESSFUL CASE STUDY

Mrs. R, a 41-year-old, married, professional businesswoman, contacted the Sleep Disorders Center in the hope that she could overcome her inability to sleep without the use of sleeping pills. Mrs. R presented as an attractive, neat, organized woman who seemed slightly anxious. She stated that her sleeping problem started eight years before when she and her first husband were having marital difficulties and he had insomnia problems. Her husband told her that her restlessness disturbed his sleep. She started taking an occasional sleeping pill to help her sleep more quietly and after three years began to use them on a regular basis. At that time, her marital difficulties had become more intense and she was in the process of divorce. Approximately three years prior to her initial visit, she became very concerned about her dependence on sleeping pills. Because of her concern, she attempted to withdraw "cold turkey," experienced two convulsions, and did not sleep at all during the three nights she was without medication. She immediately resumed taking sleeping medication (temazepam, 15 mg and oxazepam, 15 mg, before bed) and continued to do so until she sought treatment.

During the assessment, it became apparent that this woman felt most comfortable when "in control" and tended to be compulsive, organized, and somewhat of a perfectionist. She also was highly anxious about both her sleep and her dependency on medication. She was fearful about negative effects of insomnia and worried about appearing "strange" or "stupid" when sleep-deprived. She felt that if she didn't get eight hours of sleep she would not function properly at work. She was also concerned that if she had trouble sleeping, it would disturb her second husband (although he is a very good sleeper) and that ultimately her sleep problem might contribute to a failure of her second marriage. All her attempts to cope with her sleep problem had proved futile, and as a result she felt out of control, anxious, and helpless. At night, Mrs. R had trouble relaxing from her fast-paced, high-stress work environment. As bedtime approached, she would become anxious about having insomnia that night. Once in bed, Mrs. R would experience "mind racing" about work and family problems. She would become angry and upset, which would cause her to feel more aroused and more frustrated.

In setting up a treatment plan, we discussed normal sleep and the factors that influence it. Of special relevance to Mrs. R's situation was the notion of not being able to "control" sleep, but instead of setting optimal conditions for sleep to occur. We talked about events that started her cycle of insomnia, including her concern about her failing first marriage and attempts to sleep more quietly. We also identified the factors that seemed to maintain the problem, including marital difficulties, anxiety, and the use of sleeping pills.

In order to help the patient identify the specific stressors interfering with her sleep, she was told to complete a "problem diary" in the early evening between 7 and 9 P.M. She noted that working late, business deadlines, worries about her family, and stimulating conversations prior to bed all seemed to have an adverse effect on her sleep. It was helpful for her to be aware of her concerns prior to sleep and establish a new time to think about her problems other than at bedtime. She was told to keep a sleep diary and note any particularly stressful events that would affect her sleep.

Because Mrs. R had developed a negative association with her bedroom (she would be falling asleep while watching television, but when she would walk into the bedroom she would be wide awake), we started her on a modified stimulus control program. To improve her ability to relax at bedtime, she was taught deep breathing in the first session and was introduced to progressive relaxation training during the second session. She changed her evening schedule to permit adequate relaxation and "wind-down" from the day's activities. Because she was sensitive to stimulation, she limited her evening television watching to light subject matter and turned off the television completely one hour before bedtime. She found herself most relaxed if she read one hour before bedtime. She also "protected" herself by not accepting phone calls or discussing business or finances with her husband in the late evening. As a consequence, the patient reported feeling much more relaxed at bedtime. Thought stopping was introduced because of Mrs. R's difficulty with mind racing once in bed. She practiced the technique using worries about her sleep, her family, and business. She was surprised after practicing that she actually had "control" over her thoughts.

After consulting with Mrs. R's physician, a drug withdrawal program was formulated. The reduction was gradual, originally set for five weeks and later modified to take eight weeks. Her anxiety was discussed each week to give her ample opportunity to discuss her feelings and gain support from the therapist.

We discussed her fears about the effects of sleep deprivation by exploring her previous experiences when she had a bad night. Going over these issues and using cognitive restructuring to allay negative thoughts reduced her anxiety about the effects of insomnia, thereby relieving the pressure to sleep. At each meeting, we reviewed the sleep diary and focused in particular on what stress factors might have influenced a "bad" night. We also reviewed the week's "homework," eliciting her reaction to use of relaxation, stimulus control, thought stopping, and exercise. Any improvement was noted from the previous week and she was praised for her hard work and the difficult changes she had made. The treatment consisted of eight sessions and two telephone follow-ups. By the completion of treatment, Mrs. R was sleeping an average of 7.5 hours per night, falling asleep within 15 to 20 minutes, and was completely off sleeping medication.

This case study demonstrates the process by which we identified the start of Mrs. R's insomnia, the factors that maintained it, and the failure of her coping strategies. We reviewed her sleep history, and she was educated in normal sleep as well as the factors that affect it, such as the long-term use of sleeping pills. We chose intervention techniques based on the patient's particular insomnia problem, her deficiencies within the model of good sleep, her stress level, personality factors and life-style. The pace of treatment was based on her emotional skills and anxiety level. By the end of treatment, Mrs. R had a clear understanding of her sleep and had integrated positive coping strategies associated with a good night's sleep.

UNSUCCESSFUL CASE STUDY

Mrs. P, a 45-year-old married artist, sought help at the Sleep Disorders Center for her sleep-onset and maintenance insomnia. She reported that "she had had poor sleep habits since childhood but her sleep had worsened considerably over the past three or four years." This seemed to be associated with the opening of a small shop she operated with her husband. Six months previous to her visit to the Sleep Disorders Center her stress level had reached the point where she was unable to sleep at all. She was placed on triazolam, 0.25 mg, and amitriptyline, 25 mg, at bedtime by her physician. She slept fairly well, but because of her antidrug feelings she took herself off all medication and experienced rebound insomnia. After several days of not sleeping, she resumed both drugs until one week prior to her initial visit. During the previous six months her sleep had slowly deteriorated, and rather than increase her drug dosage she decided to once again stop taking medication.

The patient reported feeling very sleepy around 8:30 P.M. but after getting into bed at 9:00 P.M. would require as much as six to eight hours to fall asleep. During this time she would remain in bed and meditate and focus her attention on falling asleep. She felt that she should be able to control her sleep by focusing on making it happen. If she fell asleep, she reported awakening six to eight times and had great difficulty falling back to sleep. She estimated her total sleep time to be less than two hours every night. She would get up every morning at 7:00 A.M. and walk or run for 30 minutes. The patient reported feeling very tired in the daytime, which affected her work. She stated that "she was a very critical, demanding person and was very impatient with the fact that she couldn't sleep." The patient seemed tense and angry over her condition which she couldn't control.

The patient was educated about normal sleep and the model of a good night's sleep during the first session. It was pointed out to her that she was spending too much time in bed, and that although sleepy in the living room, she was experiencing negative conditioning to her bedroom. It was suggested that she reduce her stimulation level prior to bedtime, try to go to bed later, and use stimulus control. She was encouraged to stop trying to go to sleep and avoid meditating in bed. She was told to move her exercise time to the late afternoon.

When Mrs. P returned the following week, her sleep diary indicated a range of sleep from zero to three hours. She went to bed at 9:30 P.M., got up every morning at 7:30 A.M., avoided meditating in bed on most nights, and moved her exercise time to the late afternoon. She had difficulty in following through with stimulus control. Her husband gave her a massage every night before bed and they avoided talking about their business within an hour of bedtime. During the second week it was suggested that she keep a problem diary in the early evening after exercising. She was to write down her problems concerning work and sleep, with possible solutions. She was to get up and add to it during her sleep time if she experienced "mind racing." Because of her resistance to stimulus control, we did not further press her to do the exercise, but suggested modified sleep restriction. She was to go to bed no earlier than 10:00 P.M. and then move her bedtime later in 15-minute increments each night until she fell asleep rapidly. Time was spent in the session helping the patient better organize her time at work after her husband indicated how stressed she had become running their shop. She was given a progressive relaxation tape, which she was to practice daily.

One week later the patient reported by phone that she was still going to bed at 9:00 P.M. and had not slept at all the last two nights. Once again it was reinforced that she rest on the couch in the living room and stay out of bed until at least 10:00 P.M. She tried the relaxation tape on only two occasions but thought it was beneficial. She agreed at this point to a nocturnal polysomnogram to verify what might be disturbing her sleep. Ten days later the patient canceled her sleep recording, claiming to be sleeping much better (3 to 3.5 hours per night). She stated that she was now resting on her living room couch until after 11:00 P.M. before going to bed. Her daytime tiredness was much improved. Although she was encouraged to finish treatment, she didn't feel she needed further help from the Sleep Disorders Center.

Nothing was heard from Mrs. P for 18 months. She called once again, stating that she had slept poorly for several weeks and "wished to have an all-night sleep recording to find out what's wrong." She was taking no sedative medications. On the night of her recording she reported on her bedtime questionnaire that she had slept about two hours the previous night. The next morning the patient reported that she hadn't slept at all.

The evaluation of her sleep parameters revealed a total time in bed of seven hours, total sleep time of 4.8 hours, and a sleep efficiency of 68 percent. Latency to stage I sleep was 12 minutes, to stage II sleep 20 minutes, and to rapid-eye-movement sleep 78 minutes. She was awake for a total of two hours during her sleep period. The longest waking episodes were 16 and 66 minutes. She had six awakenings between one and ten minutes in length. It was interesting to note that her deep sleep (stage 3 to 4) was twice that expected for her age (66 minutes, 23 percent). No apnea, hypopnea, oxygen desaturation, or nocturnal myoclonus was noted. Some alpha electroencephalographic (EEG) instrusions into sleep were found.

During the interview following her all-night sleep recording, the patient steadfastly refused to believe she had slept at all. She accepted none of the explanations for her misperception of her state of consciousness, including the waking EEG intrusion into sleep or her above-normal number of awakenings greater than one minute. She felt that nocturnal polysomnograms were invalid tests of sleep. She refused all further treatment and did not follow up on two referrals to other sleep specialists in the area.

This case study demonstrates how we determine and then modify treatment strategies as the course of treatment progresses. This case points out the delicate balance between encouraging a difficult, highly anxious patient to continue an uncomfortable intervention, such as stimulus control, versus finding a "better fit," such as a highly modified sleep restriction. The case also points out how patients may leave treatment too quickly before truly integrating necessary coping strategies. They may then easily relapse.

DISCUSSION

Our treatment program for chronic insomnia focuses on selecting an optimal treatment strategy for patients by assessing as many relevant variables as possible. Our system works best with patients who can accurately report their sleep–wake history, who can reasonably perceive their own conscious states, who are able to comprehend, assimilate, and accept our model of a good night's sleep, and who understand and are motivated to do the exercises required of them. We attempt to increase compliance by encouraging patients to participate in a dialogue with us at all points during their treatment. Our effort is aimed at introducing to patients a new frame of reference for why they can't sleep, as well as to techniques that correct their unique problem. In the case of Mrs. P, our system of treatment was unsuccessful because she probably always misperceived her sleep state. Her rigid belief system allowed little opportunity for any education in good sleep hygiene or any other treatment intervention. Attempts at dialogue with the patient concerning her treatment frequently were met with an argumentative response.

We are likely to be unsuccessful with patients who, in spite of our best efforts, do not understand how someone goes about sleeping better. Patients who are intellectually impaired or with whom communication or language difficulties exist may not be able to understand the exercises they must do to improve their sleep. Sometimes a friend or family member who accompanies the patient can be of help. At home, however, without the cooperation of the patient prognosis is poor.

Some patients understand how to do a specific technique (i.e., stimulus control) but can't comprehend how doing it will help them sleep better. Sometimes creatively placing a technique within the patients' frame of reference or changing techniques to one more closely aligned with what they believe about their sleep will be helpful. For example, many patients complaining of insomnia believe that the more time they spend attempting to sleep, the more likely they are to get the sleep they need. Most patients eventually grasp the concept of negative conditioning to the bedroom and the act of sleeping and begin limiting their time in bed awake. Some stubbornly stick to their belief against all evidence to the contrary. Changing tactics by having patients sleep in a different place or by having them focus on trying to stay awake may help.

Because of the effort required on the part of the patients and because of the discomfort involved, some avoid doing the required exercises. They maintain familiar and predictable modes of inducing sleep even though they have rarely worked to solve their sleep problem in the past. This is particularly true for exercises such as stimulus control or sleep restriction, where patients may be unwilling to experience short-term pain for long-term gain. In the case of Mrs. P, she displayed minimal compliance with stimulus control and any attempts to modify her length of time in bed, stating that she was "just too tired to stay out of bed." In many patients, moving their bedtimes 15 minutes later per night will increase compliance, but even this did not work immediately for Mrs. P. Some patients become so hopelessly demoralized by their insomnia that they don't believe they are capable of modifying their sleep. These patients often leave after one session when no easy "miracle cure" is available.

Occasionally we find relatives, friends, or other professionals who are not supportive of our program and sabotage efforts by the patient to improve their sleep. A spouse who refuses to stop watching television in the bedroom or who engages in confrontational conversation with the patient just prior to bedtime makes it difficult for a patient to make headway. The patient's physician may recommend medication before our program has had a chance to work. The patient immediately sleeps better and loses the motivation to change the underlying reasons for the insomnia.

Improvement from using our model of short-term insomnia treatment is less likely with patients exhibiting certain psychiatric disorders. Patients with personality disorders who improve little even in long-term psychotherapy are poor candidates for our techniques. They fail in most aspects of what is required to succeed. These individuals have a need to maintain the safety and certainly of the status quo. Even though their insomnia symptoms are negative, they feel that if they improve their sleep they may experience even greater discomfort. Patients with avoidant personality tendencies may, for example, use insomnia to avoid many life experiences which they fear. These may include a job with more prestige or responsibility, a romantic relationship, or an educational opportunity. The patient states that they avoid these experiences because of their fears that the added stress will wreck havoc with their sleep. However, much of their avoidance is more properly due to the fear of failure of the activity itself.

Michael Stevenson is a licensed psychologist and the Clinical Director of the North Valley Sleep Disorders Center in Mission Hills, California. He has been involved in sleep research since 1973 and sleep disorders medicine since 1981. He has been accredited as a Clinical Polysomnographer by the American Sleep Disorders Association since 1983. He established one of the first Insomnia Clinics in America at Holy Cross Medical Center in Mission Hills, California, in 1983. His insomnia program has treated over 500 patients.

Marsha Weinstein is a licensed clinical social worker in private practice and an associate at North Valley Sleep Disorders Center, where she helped develop the insomnia treatment program with Dr. Stevenson and has treated over 100 insomnia patients since 1985.

RECOMMENDED READINGS

Kryger, M. H., Roth, T., & Dement, W. C. (1989). *Principles and practice of sleep medicine*. Philadelphia: W. B. Saunders, pp. 431–493.
   The insomnia section, written by several authors, covers the etiology and treatment of transient insomnias, primary insomnia, and insomnias associated with circadian rhythm disorders, psychiatric disturbances, medical disorders, and other sleep disorders.

Mendelson, W. B. (1987). Chronic insomnia. In W. B. Mendelson, *Human sleep, research and clinical care*. New York: Plenum Press, pp. 323–342.
   This chapter focuses on research into the experiences and subjective perceptions of sleep in insomniacs as well as a review of treatment approaches that have been found to be effective.

Ulene, A., & Stevenson, M. M. (1987). *How to fall asleep and stay asleep*. New York: Random House Audiobooks.
   This is a self-help audiobook for patients with insomnia. It contains interviews with insomniacs who have overcome their sleeping problems and techniques patients can use to prevent and relieve insomnia.

REFERENCES

American Psychiatric Association. (1987). *Diagnostic and statistical manual of mental disorders* (3rd ed., rev.). Washington, DC: American Psychiatric Association.

American Sleep Disorders Association Diagnostic Classification Steering Committee (Thorpy, M. J., Chairman). (1990) *The international classification of sleep disorders, diagnostic and coding manual*. Lawrence, Kansas: Allen Press.

Bootzin, R. R., & Nicassio, P. M. (1978). Behavioral treatments for insomnia. In M. Hersen, R. M. Eisler, & P. M. Miller (Eds.), *Progress in behavior modification* (Vol. 6). New York: Academic Press, pp. 1–45.

Carskadon, M. A., Dement, W. C., Mittler, M. M., Guilleminault, C., Zarcone, V. P., & Spiegel, R. (1976). Self reports versus sleep laboratory findings in 122 drug free subjects with complaints of chronic insomnia. *American Journal of Psychiatry, 133*, 1382–1383.

Curatolo, P. W., & Robertson, D. (1983). The health consequences of caffeine. *Annals of Internal Medicine, 98*, 641–653.

Czeisler, C. A., Richardson, G. S., Coleman, R. M., Zimmerman, J. C., Moore-Ede, M. C., Dement, W. C., & Weitzman, E. D. (1981). Chronotherapy: Resetting the circadian clocks of patients with delayed sleep phase insomnia. *Sleep, 4*, 1–21.

Dinges, D. F. (1989). The influence of the human circadian time keeping system on sleep. In M. H. Kryger, T. Roth, & W. C. Dement (Eds.), *Principles and practice of sleep medicine*. Philadelphia: W. B. Saunders, pp. 153–162.

Hoddes, E., Zarcone, V. P., Smythe, H., Phillips, R., & Dement, W. C. (1973). Quantification of sleepiness: A new approach. *Psychophysiology, 10*, 431–436.

Horne, J. (1988). *Why we sleep: The functions of sleep in humans and other mammals.* Oxford: Oxford University Press.
Horne, J. A., & Porter, J. M. (1976). Time of day effects with standardized exercise upon subsequent sleep. *Electroencephalography and Clinical Neurophysiology, 40,* 178–184.
Jacobson, E. (1974). *Progressive relaxation.* Chicago: University of Chicago Press.
Mahoney, M. J. (1974). *Cognition and behavior modification.* Cambridge, MA: Ballinger.
McMullen, R. E. (1986). *Handbook of cognitive therapy techniques.* New York: W. W. Norton.
Nicholson, A. N. (1989). Hypnotics: Clinical pharmacology and therapeutics. In M. H. Kryger, T. Roth, & W. C. Dement (Eds.), *Principles and practice of sleep medicine.* Philadelphia: W. B. Saunders, pp. 219–227.
Reynolds, C. F., Kupfer, D. J., Taska, L. S., Hoch, C. C., Sewitch, D. E., & Spiker, D. G. (1985). The sleep of health seniors: A revisit. *Sleep, 8,* 20–29.
Smith, J. C. (1985). *Relaxation dynamics: Nine world approaches to self-relaxation.* Champaign, IL: Research Press.
Soldatos, C. R., Kales, J. D., Scharf, M. B., Bixler, E. O., & Kales, A. (1980). Cigarette smoking associated with sleep difficulty. *Science, 207,* 551–552.
Spielman, A. J., Saskin, P., & Thorpy, M. J. (1987). Treatment of chronic insomnia by restriction of time in bed. *Sleep, 10,* 45–56.
Zarcone, V. P. (1989). Sleep hygiene. In M. H. Kryger, T. Roth, & W. C. Dement, (Eds.), *Principles and practice of sleep medicine.* Philadelphia: W. B. Saunders, pp. 490–493.

CHAPTER TEN

Breaking the Vicious Circle of Insomnia
A Treatment Model

NEIL STEINBERG

INTRODUCTION

Intense psychological pain and a major disruption of daily life invariably accompany chronic insomnia. These patients feel an urgent need for help. Fear and anger, in response to not controlling sleep, often lead to feelings of powerlessness, despair, and increasing frustration. Unfortunately, these emotional reactions are instrumental in transforming transient insomnia into chronic insomnia. Emotional stress occasionally brings transient sleeplessness to almost everyone; however, an intense emotional reaction to sleeplessness combines with conditioning or learning patterns to perpetuate temporary sleeplessness into agonizing and life-disruptive chronic insomnia.

The sleep–wake cycle is a natural human process. A disruption of this natural cycle presents a clear message that the person's thoughts, emotions, and/or behavior need to change so the natural propensity to sleep returns. The emotional reaction to chronic insomnia necessitates that the clinician remind the patient that sleep is a natural process. Chronic insomniacs often suffer in attempts to force themselves to sleep. Ironically, these efforts only perpetuate their sleeplessness. It is crucial that insomniacs learn to identify ways in which they are disrupting their own natural sleep patterns and, with clinical assistance, remove these disruptions.

Insomnia treatment largely focuses on removing experiences, behav-

---

Neil Steinberg • Clinical Sleep Services, Santa Rosa, California 95402.

iors, and environmental factors blocking the natural sleep–wake balance. Insomnia forms a self-perpetuating vicious circle. Each component of this circle must be identified and multiple treatments sequentially introduced in order to break this vicious, self-perpetuating pattern. Each treatment intervention aims at removing the blockage of the person's natural ability to sleep.

BACKGROUND

For many years I joined the majority of my psychologist and psychiatrist colleagues in interpreting insomnia as a symptom of depression or anxiety. I too held the view that insomnia does not require treatment, but rather that, as the depression and anxiety recede, so will the insomnia. For several years I observed that this causal relationship often did not exist, yet I continued to convince myself that insomnia did not need to be a focus of treatment. Finally, after several years of this clinical folly, I began to research the phenomenon and potential treatment approaches for this sleep disorder. I was relieved to find confirmation of what I had observed to be true for many years—that insomnia *is* a distinct condition.

As I pursued the research and theoretical literature on the evaluation and treatment of insomnia, I was impressed with the various psychophysiological, behavioral, and psychotherapeutic approaches to this pioneering area of sleep disorder treatment.

The primary insomnia treatment approaches presented in the research and theoretical literature include *stimulus control* (Bootzin & Nicassio, 1978; Haynes *et al.*, 1975); *cognitive restructuring* (Thoresen *et al.*, 1981); *progressive relaxation* (Jacobson, 1938; Lazarus, 1976); *biofeedback* (Hauri *et al.*, 1982); *reciprocal inhibition* (Evans & Bond, 1969); *autogenic training* (Ribordy & Denney, 1977); *paradoxical intention* (Frankl, 1960; Ascher & Turner, 1978); *restricted time in bed* (Spielman *et al.*, 1987); *supportive and explorative psychotherapy* (Soldatos *et al.*, 1979; Kales & Kales, 1984); and *cognitive focusing* (Woolfolk *et al.*, 1976).

These various treatments demonstrate significant levels of effectiveness in treating chronic insomnia. Each approach contributes to alleviating this sleep disorder. I, however, found it surprising that most of these treatment interventions do not acknowledge the effectiveness of other approaches nor do they attempt to create integrated models of resolving this condition. Turner and Ascher (1979) conducted a controlled comparison of progressive relaxation, stimulus control, and paradoxical intention therapies for insomnia. Their research indicates that these three treatments separately produced significantly greater improvement of sleep that the nontreatment control group. Thus a myriad of treatment forms offer effective intervention for insomnia. A comprehensive, integrated insomnia treatment model is needed so the contributions of various treatment approaches can be combined in a mutually beneficial manner to offer the patient optimal, full-range insomnia treatment.

METHOD

The vicious circle of insomnia (see Figure 1, inner circle) typically begins with incidents of emotional upset and acute stress. These experiences, in turn, create physiological tension and arousal and, consequently, insomnia. At this point, the person often feels tension and anxiety when preparing for bed and spends time in bed engaging in nonsleep activities and worry, behaviors that are contradictory to sleep. By pairing these nonsleep and countersleep behaviors with bed and bedtime, the individual begins to unwittingly learn sleeplessness. This condition is referred to as a learned dysfunctional sleep pattern. The sleeplessness thus continues, and the insomniac further develops fear and anger in response to not sleeping. Greater emotional upset occurs, and the vicious circle of insomnia is set in motion. Without intervention, this circle of dysfunctional sleep often persists for many years.

The outer circle of Figure 1 shows the treatment approaches and the points of the vicious circle of insomnia to which they are applied. This comprehensive, integrated treatment model incorporates contributions of various treatment approaches and acknowledges the central role of emotions and psychotherapeutic intervention.

Prior to the initial appointment, I send the patient an insomnia treatment patient questionnaire. At the first appointment we review the questionnaire responses to determine the type, duration, severity, and causes of the insomnia. This shows which aspects of the patient's vicious circle of insomnia are most in need of intervention and which treatments are most applicable to this person's insomnia.

Upon completing the questionnaire review, I conduct a structured intake interview. Answers to the questions describe the two hours before going to bed on the night prior to the first treatment session. Often insomniacs struggle to generalize about their before-bed behaviors, but when asked specifically about the prior night, they describe their behaviors accurately. The origin of the insomnia and relevant personal history follow. I review the current nature of the person's insomnia. I ask the patient again about the current pattern of sleeplessness to further elucidate information presented on the insomnia questionnaire. As shown on the

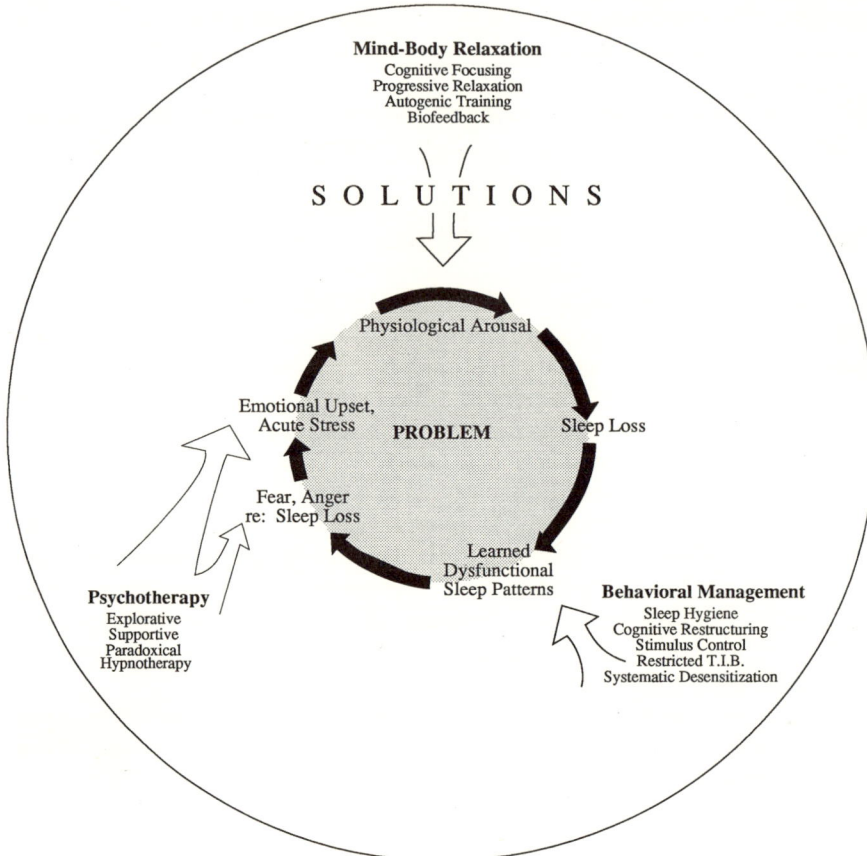

Figure 1. (Inner portion) The vicious circle of insomnia. (Outer Portion) The treatments which break this painful circle and often stop the sleeplessness. Medical treatment is integrated wth this model when physical ailments or drugs are a source of the insomnia, and in some cases in which short-term, intermittent sleep medication is a treatment adjunct. (Copyright © 1990 Clinical Sleep Services.)

intake sheet, I then begin to evaluate the patient for conditioned or learned sleeplessness resulting from the association of bedroom and bed with nonsleep behavior. This section of questions also clarifies the significance of the person's emotional reaction to not sleeping as a central element of his circle of insomnia.

Exploration of the patient's perspective of his sleeplessness is next. The patient's self-description and hypotheses about his insomnia begin to exhibit the psychological component of the insomnia, specifically the tendency to suppress and internalize emotions, depression, obsessive compulsiveness, and interpersonal problems. The patient often begins to discuss mind–body stress and tension as components of insomnia, as well as the thoughts and self-dialogue that perpetuate the sleeplessness. Before behavioral, mind–body, or psychotherapeutic treatments are pursued, it is crucial to rule out physiological illness or conditions as primary causes of the insomnia. For example, if the patient experiences nocturnal myoclonus, uncomfortable and disruptive leg movement and sensations, or apnea, referrals for a polysomnograph laboratory test or examination by an appropriate physician are required.

Frequently the insomniac patient experiences an urgency for help and clearly communicates, either verbally or nonverbally, the desire for immediate interventions and treatments. However, it is my experience that initially it is important to proceed slowly and cautiously. Often, two or even three sessions are necessary to comprehensively diagnose the nature of the patient's insomnia before treatments are introduced. Premature and inappropriate introduction of psychotherapeutic, behavioral, or mind–body interventions can sabotage effective treatment and further contribute to the patient's feelings of despair and isolation regarding his insomnia. During this diagnostic period it is important to reassure the patient that we will likely make significant progress in reducing and eliminating the insomnia, but it is crucial that we begin slowly. At this stage of treatment it is helpful to begin sleep hygiene evaluation and education (Hauri, 1982) regarding regularity of sleep schedules, exercise, sleep environment, noise and temperature, eating and consumption of alcohol, caffeine, and nicotine.

Upon completion of the structured intake interview, I question the patient about particular areas that stand out as especially problematic in his or her own vicious circle of insomnia. For example, if physical tension is particularly intense and troublesome at bedtime, I ask in detail about the general stress/tension level, evening activities, and physical and emotional experiences while both preparing for and in bed.

Figure 1 illustrates the categories of treatment and points of intervention. Each treatment category aims at removing a barrier blocking the natural sleep–wake cycle. The psychotherapeutic treatments help reduce and resolve the emotional reaction to sleeplessness and, in some cases, the psychological causes of the insomnia. Such emotions impede the return of natural sleep rhythm. The mind–body relaxation treatments reduce the physiological overactivation and tension that stop natural sleep physiology and the necessary quieting of thoughts. Occasionally, short-term intermittent sleep medication enables the person to sleep, reducing the frustration and fear that prevent the return of a healthy sleep pattern. Potential dependency, memory loss, and rebound effects of such medication require careful evaluation of such pharmacological interventions. Behavior management approaches utilize conditioning and social learning to reassociate bedtime and bed with sleep. Inadvertent learning of insomnia blocks sleep–wake health and must be conditioned to reconstruct a positive sleep pattern. These various categories of treatment are interdependent. Use of more than one type of treatment is typically necessary for effective, lasting treatment.

It is my consistent experience with chronic insomniacs that their emotional reaction to sleeplessness is often the most significant single component of their vicious circle of insomnia. Fear, anger, and shame are the most powerful binding aspects of this self-perpetuating pathology. Consequently, psychotherapeutic approaches frequently comprise a major sphere of the interventions that most effectively reduce and eliminate the insomnia. The application of psychotherapy for chronic insomnia has been questioned because of the limited ability and willingness of most patients to participate in such insight-oriented exploration and because the emotionally upsetting precipitating causes of insomnia are often either resolved or not consciously accessible to the patient. The psychotherapeutic interventions aimed at the emotional response to sleeplessness, rather than treating the initial emotional precipitating causes of the insomnia, typically provide the greatest assistance. Often these feelings are sufficiently available to the patient's consciousness to be relatively easily facilitated by the clinician. As these traumas remain unresolved, conscious, and painfully current, the patient frequently exhibits sufficient motivation and insight to progress psychotherapeutically.

Major life-stress events and intense emotional upset result in sleeplessness for most people. As the stress and upset subside, normal sleep typically returns. However, certain psychological predispositions characterize people whose healthy sleep patterns do not return when trauma and stress subside. The primary psychological characteristics distinguishing chronic from short-term insomniacs include internalizing rather than expressing emotions, a heightened need for control, isolation resulting from emotional and/or social withdrawal, obsession–compulsion patterns, interpersonal difficulties, and substantial discontent with past and present family and health experiences. Much of the discussion of psychotherapeutic interventions in this chapter focuses on the specific distinguishing traits of chronic insomniacs. These psychological characteristics frequently impede the return of healthy sleep patterns. Psychotherapeutic interventions aimed at altering these personality factors and coping mechanisms, at least as they relate to the person's sleep behaviors and reactions to sleeplessness, are frequently instrumental in producing lasting effective treatment.

I encourage the patient to become increasingly aware of his or her emotions in response to not sleeping. Most patients quickly become aware of strong feelings and are encouraged to begin describing and expressing these feelings. As many insomniacs internalize their emotions by denying and suppressing feelings, a fair amount of patience and skill by the clinician to facilitate expression of such feelings is required. Intense emotions chronically suppressed during the day tend to intrude on the person's awareness at night, creating tension and agitation.

Emotional expression is often quite important so that the insomniac can begin to reduce the physiological charge resulting from the suppressed emotion and the resultant tension and agitation. Such expression also frequently enables more effective application of behavioral treatment approaches. Unexpressed intense emotions related to sleep greatly hinder lasting effectiveness through mind–body relaxation and behavioral learning techniques. Helping the patient identify and discharge his or her intense emotional response to sleeplessness often contributes to the success of other types of treatment.

A circularity to the effectiveness of the various areas of insomnia treatment is apparent. As mind–body relaxation and behavioral management treatments, such as progressive relaxation, stimulus control, and cognitive restructuring, are applied with effectiveness, the patient's sleep improves, reducing the charge of the emotional reaction to not sleeping. The improving sleep often leads to increased awareness of the emotional reactions to not sleeping and to feeling safer in expressing such feelings. Likewise, as emotions are identified and expressed psychotherapeutically, the behavioral treatment's success is facilitated. Frequently, all areas of treatment for this condition contribute to, support, and increase the prognosis of other treatments being presented simultaneously or in sequence.

The therapeutic alliance between the clinician and the patient is a powerful aspect of the treatment. Isolation and powerlessness represent much of the psychological pain of insomniacs. As withdrawal and a heightened need for control typify many chronic insomniacs, these responses to sleeplessness are predictable. The partnership between the clinician and the patient greatly contributes to reduction of the insomniac's isolation and powerlessness, thus often providing a central ingredient of successful treatment.

A SUCCESSFUL CASE

David is a 12-year-old boy whose mother requested treatment of his insomnia, "bad nightmares," and sleepwalking. I sent him a patient questionnaire. David's mother accompanied him for the first visit. Review of the questionnaire clarified David's severe difficulty with both getting to sleep and remaining asleep. David frequently required 45 minutes to an hour to fall asleep and then often awakened during the night for one- to two-hour periods. This pattern had become upsetting to David and his parents.

I selected this case because of David's willingness and ability to present himself in a very honest, innocent manner. Self-disclosure is frequently compromised by adult patients' denial and self-consciousness. David exemplifies and elucidates many of the common central dynamics of insomniacs of all ages.

The intake interview demonstrated that David began to feel fearful and anxious approximately an hour before his bedtime, increasingly fearing not sleeping. He also described that upon awakening, his first thought was "You're not going to be able to sleep." "Go upstairs and be with your parents" often followed as his next thought.

Regarding the origin of his insomnia, when David was six his brother, with whom he had been sharing a bedroom, moved into another room in the house, and David began sleeping alone. Both he and his mother remembered this as the time when David developed difficulties getting to sleep and staying asleep. Though he had sought and received counseling and attempted hypnotherapy for insomnia, his symptoms remained unaltered.

When I asked David what made him sleep better or worse, he stated that nothing made it better and that he frequently became angry at himself for not controlling his sleep. He further said, "I go to my parents' room and sleep in a sleeping bag. I don't remember going there a lot of the time, but I remember sleeping good." At the end of the initial session, David sought suggestions or remedies for his insomnia. I asked him if he would be patient and wait a week before we attempted to solve his problem. I assured him that it was quite likely that his sleep would improve and that most people who receive insomnia treatment learn to sleep substantially better. He expressed relief that his mother had finally found someone who knew how to help people who could not sleep.

At the next session, David told me how angry he had been feeling at himself for not sleeping. When he woke up in the night and could not quickly return to sleep, he became very angry and agitated. He began to realize that his self-anger was in response to knowing he was worrying his parents. We discussed the importance he placed on pleasing his parents and his awareness of their level of fear and worry about his inability to sleep. At this point I spoke to David about the incompatibility of anger and sleep. He grasped how his anger led to physiological arousal and resulted in wakefulness.

David understood this emotion–body relationship and expressed interest in learning how to change his self-defeating pattern. I then instructed David on the method of progressive relaxation. I spent the second half of this session teaching him how to systematically tense and then release and relax the various muscle groups of his body. I also gave him an audio cassette tape with which to practice during the day for three or four days. Then, if he was gaining comfort and confidence in his ability to follow the progressive relaxation instructions, he was to use it at bedtime and during nocturnal awakenings when he started to become angry at himself. He expressed optimism about reducing his anger in this way.

We agreed that the next week I would spend time separately with David's mother and father to address their fear in response to David's insomnia. David is hypervigilant and responsive to their upset about him. The parents needed assistance in learning to relax and resolve their upset about David's insomnia.

When David began his next session, he vividly exhibited agitation with himself. He expressed his frustration in response to "failing" the progressive relaxation training. He had used this technique each day during the week since he last saw me but became increasingly tense in the process. He felt impatient with his lack of success but proceeded to use it at bedtime and during nocturnal awakenings. This treatment attempt intensified his insomnia rather than reduced it. I explained to David that there are many approaches we could use, and we did not have to work so hard at succeeding with a particular approach that did not seem to work. I also again discussed the importance of limiting his anger toward himself when he was attempting to sleep.

I asked David if he would be interested in trying a different approach to see if we would have more success. He was eager to try. I spent the remainder of the session teaching him autogenic training, a process of self-suggestion to relax the body and autonomic nervous system. Through my systematically suggesting that he experience the various parts of his body as heavy and warm, he began to feel relaxation and quieting of his thoughts. I presented this mind–body relaxation treatment in the context of David's learning to reduce the tension and self-anger that interfere with his natural sleep–wake cycle. He was more receptive to the autogenic training than the progressive relaxation. It was not completely clear why this technique was more effective. Possibly the simplicity and body sensation orientation provided the essential elements. However, knowing which treatments help is more crucial than knowing why they help. When he practiced the tape-recorded autogenic training on his own during the following week, he relaxed a great deal and experienced reduced anger at night. This technique helped with getting to sleep and also when he woke up and began to feel anger toward himself in response to awakening.

In the session with the parents, we began to explore their fear and feelings of powerlessness in attempting to help David with his severe chronic insomnia. In recent discussions with David, it had become increasingly clear that much of their son's upset was in response to their own emotional reactions. We discussed the importance of learning to utilize each other in an effort to reduce and resolve their own feelings of fear about David's insomnia. They also had begun to realize that David was not upset by his "nightmares" but, in fact, rarely remembered either his "nightmares" or walking and talking in his sleep. The parents had assumed that these were traumatic experiences for David but were discovering that only they were upset. These were night terrors, and they did not seem to have residual upsetting effects on David.

During the night terrors David approached his parents while still asleep and described very traumatic experiences. However, the next morning he neither recalled nor felt any aftereffects from these experiences. Throughout the remainder of his insomnia treatment, the parents periodically participated in sessions with me. They continued to resolve their own upset so as not to contribute to his insomnia difficulties. Intervention with family members is often helpful in insomnia treatment. The response of other family members to the insomniac's behavior often unwittingly contributes to perpetuation of this condition.

Continued success with autogenic training led to a reduction of self-anger and an improvement of sleep. David began gaining confidence in his ability to reconstruct a positive sleep pattern. Feeling "in control of his sleep" had eluded David for the past six years. We explored his perfectionism and need to please others. David perceived with increasing clarity his limited tolerance for making mistakes. His perfectionism appeared to enter every aspect of his life, including school, sports, relationships, and his ability to sleep. He expressed his response to imperfection by exerting increasing control on himself. One of the personality characteristics common to many chronic insomniacs is a heightened need for control. This is frequently an aspect of the person's response to sleep which requires psychotherapeutic attention as part of the insomnia treatment.

Although many patients may not be interested in long-term insight-oriented psychotherapy, they are nonetheless often open to exploring specifically their control needs and behaviors as they relate to insomnia patterns. As chronic insomnia is an extremely psychologically painful condition, a high level of motivation and willingness to explore oneself, at least with a specific focus, is often present. Thus, I began exploring with David his need for and efforts to control his sleep. I utilized the autogenic training as a way of describing how he ironically "gained control" of his sleep by releasing his typical attempts to control himself. By relaxing his body and thoughts he began to invite sleep and not disrupt the natural sleep–wake process by exerting attempts to directly control sleep. I again reminded David that sleep is a natural experience, and all he needed to do was learn not to disrupt what his mind and body naturally seek.

Over the next few weeks David remained focused on his impulses to control his sleep and force himself to go to sleep. He also showed increased awareness of how his need to control feeds his physiological and mental arousal, leading to insomnia. By exploring and expressing his frustration, self-anger, and need to control his sleep, he began to relinquish these efforts to force himself to sleep. Expressions of these feelings during the day led to their reduction at night. Like many insomniacs, David was unfamiliar with expressing his emotions. The way in which he silently became angry and self-controlling typified his personality and the personalities of many chronic insomniacs. He continued to understand how his emotional upset, especially when unexpressed, would lead to physiological arousal and further sleeplessness. This boy's response to not sleeping created the center of his emotional upset.

David began to understand and resolve his self-destructive pattern of suppressing his emotional expressions. His predominantly quiet, contemplative, cautious nature began to yield to exploration and expression of emotions in his treatment. On certain nights, when it was clear to him that he was angry with himself and attempting to control behaviors, he was taught to get out of bed and write his angry and controlling thoughts and feelings in a sleep journal. This led to more rapid resolution of his anger and a reduction in the length of his nocturnal awakening. Getting out of bed when he was angry also prevented the association of bed and agitation and subsequent learned or conditioned insomnia. On most nights, however, he continued to utilize the autogenic training and prevents his anger and agitation through this process.

In subsequent treatment sessions with David individually and with his mother, it became increasingly clear that his insomnia was, in part, a response to feelings of loss and isolation. The first clue was the inception of his insomnia when he began to sleep alone in a bedroom. The next indicator of the significance of isolation was his urgent need that his father become more involved in his insomnia treatment. David expressed feeling abandoned by his father's limited interaction with him in his daily life. He spoke of specific upset regarding his father's apparent disinterest in his son's insomnia trauma and treatment. I then began to involve his father in more of the treatment sessions and encouraged the father to express his interest in and increase his interaction with his son, especially regarding the sleep disturbance. Though the father was privately concerned about his son, he infrequently expressed such concern and rarely asked his son about the insomnia difficulties. The father typically would gain information from the mother, leaving the son unaware of his father's concern.

During the past year, David's older brother was killed in a motorcycle accident. David's feelings of isolation and abandonment related to this loss were filled with deep pain. Often insomniacs feel a great deal of emotional pain in regard to isolation with their insomnia. They feel very alone in this condition and often are emotionally withdrawn from others. As mentioned earlier, chronic insomniacs frequently suppress their feelings and internalize the expression of their emotions, thus leaving them further withdrawn and isolated. Much of David's feelings and patterns typify many insomniacs. Thus, he was encouraged to talk about his sleep problems much more with his family. I encouraged the expression of his emotions about his sleeplessness, not only to me but to his mother and father. David, his mother, and his father participated in joint sessions, specifically focusing on his feelings of isolation. I encouraged them to share their mutual insomnia fears and frustrations. These interventions appeared to be productive, and in subsequent sessions David verbalized relief in not experiencing the insomnia alone. He also was visibly pleased with his father's interest and involvement in his sleep disturbance. This type of family involvement also applies to treatment of adult insomnia. Family members and close friends often contribute to the insomnia treatment. The interactions between insomniacs and other important people in their lives tend to perpetuate rather than eliminate symptoms. In this case the parents' upset resulted in David's self-anger, and the father's unexpressed concerns for David led to David's increased feelings of isolation.

David diligently charted his daily bedtime and sleep behavior in a sleep log. During the first eight weeks of his treatment the log showed his sleep consistently improving. He gained confidence in his ability to reconstruct his natural sleep–wake pattern gradually and consistently. He continued to utilize the autogenic training, his journal writing, and discussions with his family. I continued to encourage him to identify and express his emotions, both in session and with his family, regarding his sleep difficulties. He eventually channeled his control needs away from attempting to force himself to sleep. Sleep performance anxiety and subsequent physiological arousal in response to his sleeplessness decreased.

David now sleeps eight hours per night, with normal awakenings. I discussed with him discontinuing treatment. Initially he felt fearful that he could not maintain his improved sleep if he did not continue to see me. He felt that I had taken away his insomnia and that if he discontinued his relationship with me, the insomnia would return. The therapeutic alliance I had formed with David was central to his treatment success. Our relationship enabled him to break his emotional isolation and helped him regain a sense of control and power related to his sleep. Thus discontinuing treatment was frightening to him.

It was agreed that we gradually lengthen the time between his sessions so he could step by step test his ability to maintain his sleep without me. Initially, when sleeplessness returned, he attributed his insomnia to the length of time since he had seen me. However, over the next few weeks his sleep improvement strengthened, and he gradually shifted the attribution of his improved sleep from me to himself.

David's age contributed to his willingness to openly and innocently describe his treatment experiences, which typified those of all ages. An example of this clarity was his description of feeling dependent on me. He continued seeing me monthly for three months. We then agreed that he would telephone for an appointment if he experienced a recurrence of his insomnia. After six months he called for an appointment. After one session he felt able to return to the techniques and behavior he had learned with me. Following that incident, for the last year and a half he has maintained his improved sleep behavior. The entire family expresses great relief that this source of upset has finally exited from their lives.

UNSUCCESSFUL CASE

A 35-year-old single woman, Tricia, described herself on the patient questionnaire as experiencing long-term difficulties getting to sleep and remaining asleep. This insomnia had been a serious problem for the past eight years. She admitted poor sleep hygiene, namely, her consumption of alcohol in the evening and caffeine during the day. Tricia indicated that she spent substantial periods in bed nightly engaged in nonsleep activities, including reading, watching television, and worrying. In addition to emotional upset regarding her sleep, she described a great deal of dissatisfaction regarding her love relationships and sex life. Her fear of not falling asleep was her most intense emotional difficulty.

In response to my questions using the sleep and personal history intake sheet, Tricia stated that her intense fears about sleeping frequently began sometime in the midafternoon. She often became increasingly tense and agitated in anticipation of not sleeping. She greatly feared not being able to get to sleep. Ironically, she also consistently experienced anger that she needed to end her day by sleeping. She stated, "Then I have to go into myself, be alone, focus on my feelings. I dislike having to arbitrarily cut off my activities and go to bed and be all alone."

In the first session I gathered the above information and reassured Tricia that frequently people receiving formalized insomnia treatment learn to significantly improve their sleep. She was eager to receive treatment and also inquired about being referred for sleep medication. I gave her a sleep hygiene manual and began discussing with her the effects of her consumption of caffeine and alcohol. A family physician had recommended a couple of drinks of alcohol in the evening to help her sleep. She expressed surprise when I informed her that her nocturnal awakenings were probably, in part, a chemical, physiological reaction to the late-evening consumption of alcohol. I also encouraged her to reduce, if not eliminate, her consumption of caffeine. I gave Tricia a sleep log form and encouraged her to note all the nonsleep activities in which she engaged while in bed. I spoke with her briefly about the possible learning of dysfunctional sleep patterns (conditioning) that may have resulted from her nonsleep activities in bed.

The sleep log she completed between the first and second sessions further clarified her potential for conditioning her sleeplessness through the association of bedtime and bed with wakefulness-inducing, nonsleep activities. I reviewed with her the vicious circle of insomnia diagram, explaining how her sleeplessness was being unintentionally strengthened and perpetuated by associating thought and emotion-provoking activities with bed and bedtime. I then presented the stimulus control treatment (Bootzin & Nicassio, 1978) to Tricia. She was informed that the purpose of this treatment is to reassociate the bedroom stimuli with a rapid sleep-onset response, rather than a frustration and arousal response. Instructions included going to bed only when sleepy, using her bed only for sleeping, and not watching television, reading, eating, or worrying while in bed. When unable to sleep, she was asked to get out of bed, leave the bedroom, and return only when she was really sleepy. I encouraged Tricia to continue this pattern through the night and to set her alarm and get up at the same time every morning. Thus her body would begin to learn a consistent sleep–wake rhythm. I recommended the discontinuation of naps. Expressing some unhappiness and frustration with this treatment approach, she stated her willingness to participate. This resistance is not unusual for someone who is already deprived of sleep and upset about not sleeping. We spent the remainder of the session discussing her bedtime and bed behaviors and her feelings about participating in the stimulus control treatment.

At the next session we discussed Tricia's sleep hygiene behaviors, specifically consumption of alcohol and caffeine, and her experience in following the stimulus control treatment during the past week. She exhibited resistance to changing her sleep-related behaviors. Tricia had begun to make some slight behavioral changes and expressed the intention to change more fully. She acknowledged difficulty in changing her behaviors, but stated that the extreme discomfort she felt motivated her to continue working toward change. Tricia expressed interest in beginning to learn relaxation techniques which she had seen on the diagram for treatment of the vicious circle of insomnia. She experienced a great deal of physiological arousal and tension at bedtime and during the night. However, it seemed premature to introduce yet another treatment modality in view of her limited progress with the treatments already presented. I encouraged her to spend the remainder of the session further exploring her resistance to both sleep hygiene changes and implementation of the stimulus control procedures. She further agreed to continue her sleep log and recommitted to continuing the procedures designed to reassociate bedroom stimuli with the onset and maintenance of sleep.

In the next session, Tricia spoke of her strong feelings in response to two men with whom she had recently formed intimate relationships. It appeared throughout previous sessions that Tricia exhibited many of the psychological predispositions of chronic insomniacs. I agreed to enter a psychotherapeutic discussion regarding her relationships as a doorway to the personality aspects of her insomnia. A primary psychological dynamic affecting her sleeplessness was feeling forced to withdraw from others, entering the isolation of sleep. Though she frequently experienced strong emotion, she rarely expressed such feeling and often blatantly denied her emotions to others and to herself. Tricia also consistently exhibited a strong need to control her experiences and behaviors. It seemed likely that her emotional upset about her two newly formed relationships involved several of the psychological characteristics related to chronic insomnia.

To confront what appeared to be her typical pattern of internalizing emotions, I encouraged her to directly express her anger and fear in relationship to the two men she had begun to discuss at the beginning of the session. She initially denied such feelings and contended she was just worried and confused. However, with further encouragement she began to experience and express rather strong emotions. She exhibited increasing anxiety and agitation while becoming more aware of the compulsiveness and urgency of her sexual needs. At the close of the session she noted that we had not discussed her insomnia.

Prior to Tricia's subsequent session she telephoned to inform me she was discontinuing her insomnia treatment, that I had not told her anything she didn't already know, and seeing me was an obvious waste of her time and money. She further informed me that if we had just discussed her sleep difficulties, she probably would have remained in treatment. However, since she was upset by what had occurred during the last session, she absolutely refused to return and further discuss her insomnia or the continuation of her treatment.

Tricia was correct. The psychotherapeutic intervention aimed at beginning to explore and resolve issues regarding isolation and control were untimely and a therapeutic error. Her treatment was slowed by fear and resistance, but she demonstrated some progress with behavioral insomnia treatments. In hindsight, I could see she had communicated her inability and/or unwillingness to express strong emotion and psychologically explore herself. In her first session she had stated that one of the aspects of going to bed and sleep which she most deplored was experiencing her emotions. Remaining in treatment and continuing to establish progress with sleep hygiene, behavioral management, and mind–body relaxation techniques may have led to a willingness to slowly identify and express the emotional component of her insomnia.

Identification and resolution of her fear and anger in response to sleeping and not sleeping would have strengthened the effectiveness of her insomnia treatment. Emotions comprised a significant component of her vicious circle of insomnia, requiring psychotherapeutic intervention for optimal treatment. Tricia was overwhelmed by the poor timing of this intervention. Discontinuation and failure of the overall treatment resulted. Emotional reaction to both sleeping and not sleeping was the core of Tricia's vicious circle of insomnia. In addition to poor timing, explorative psychotherapeutic intervention may not have been possible at any point in her treatment. My attempt to apply this model's full range of treatment led to failure.

DISCUSSION

Optimal application of this model for treating the vicious circle of insomnia requires that the patient participate in each of the treatment components. The circularity of the symptoms and the mutual interdependency of the treatments form the basis of the model. The relaxation treatments help reduce the patient's physiological arousal, assisting him or her in more successfully engaging in behavioral treatments. Psychotherapeutic interventions assist in identifying and expressing emotion, thus reducing chronic internalization and physiological arousal resulting from failure to express feelings. Reduction of suppressed emotion facilitates the success of relaxation treatments and behavioral approaches.

Reciprocally, behavioral management interventions enable the insomniac to experience more success and control with sleep and allow the patient to become more conscious and confident with general issues of control. Consequently, he or she feels more confident and able to explore and express these psychological dynamics psychotherapeutically. The mind–body relaxation approaches also contribute to psychotherapy by allowing the patient to reduce the intensity of his or her tension and emotional charge and more comfortably explore and express such feelings. When short-term intermittent sleep medication is applied, it assists the insomniac in reducing or disrupting the intensity of the fear of not sleeping and allows him or her to more comfortably and successfully engage in each of the other treatment approaches.

This interdependency and reciprocity of treatments exhibit the primary strength of this comprehensive treatment model. The integrated treatment approach addresses the patient's sleep-related emotions, thoughts, behavior, and physiology which interrupt the natural sleep–wake balance. Each treatment aims at an aspect of the patient's vicious circle of insomnia. The patient's willingness and ability to participate in each of the applicable treatment areas enhances the likelihood of success.

The emotional response to sleeplessness frequently presents as the component most instrumental in perpetuating chronic insomnia. Thus, it is often important that the patient be willing and able to explore and reduce the destructiveness of this element of the vicious circle. Behavioral learning or conditioning also frequently comprises a major aspect of the perpetuating process. Thus, the patient's willingness to alter behaviors to strengthen the stimulus of bed and bedtime with the response of sleep becomes another important sphere of treatment success.

In the case of David, his willingness and ability to participate in all the treatment areas of the model demonstrate the strength and success of this comprehensive treatment approach. However, in the case of Tricia, she exhibited unwillingness and/or psychological inability to participate in psychotherapeutic interventions, at least in the manner and timing I introduced them in her treatment. This treatment model presented in its entirety thus is not applicable to all chronic insomniacs. As emotion is often the most binding component of the circle of insomnia, the application of this comprehensive model often focuses on psychotherapeutic interventions. If the patient is not emotionally available for exploration and expression of his or her feelings, at least in response to sleeplessness, then this treatment model in its entirety has limited application.

In the case of Tricia, the application of psychotherapy was premature, if not inappropriate. The further development of trust in her therapeutic relationship with me and the gaining of confidence through successful application of the behavioral treatment approaches may have enabled her to engage in the psychotherapeutic aspects of the treatment. However, it is possible that she would not have been receptive to such interventions regardless of the timing and sequence of treatments presented. As many chronic insomniacs internalize rather than express their emotions, the application of psychotherapy requires skill, thorough evaluation, and good timing.

Rigid application of this treatment model in its entirely will lead to failure with certain patients not amenable to certain treatment approaches. It is important that when clinicians utilize this treatment model, they recognize and accept the strengths and limitations of the patients they treat. If the insomniac shows discomfort and lacks familiarity with body sensations, progressive relaxation and autogenic training will probably not be successful, at least in earlier stages of the treatment. Exceptionally strong oppositional behavior and/or fear of control by others indicates that behavioral treatments, such as stimulus control, may not be applicable.

Few professionals at present have gained the knowledge and skill to treat the widespread and traumatic condition of insomnia effectively. Those of us providing this urgently needed treatment must remain attentive, receptive, and responsive to the ability and willingness of patients to participate in different treatment components. We need to be flexible in applying this comprehensive treatment model. If the insomniac demonstrates emotional or intellectual inability or unwillingness to utilize a certain treatment approach, it is important that we apply other treatments which may have the potential to assist in reconstructing healthy sleep patterns. Rigid and perfectionistic application of this comprehensive treatment model often results in failure. Creativity, flexibility, and responsiveness to the patient usually lead to success.

CONCLUSION

Success or failure of this treatment model depends on the knowledge, skill, and experience of the clinician to determine which elements of the patient's vicious circle of insomnia most need intervention and change and to what extent that particular insomniac is willing and able to respond. The clinician must become skilled in the full range of treatments or refer the patient for specific treatment components, carefully and completely coordinate the treatments, and assist the patient in utilizing and integrating these various interventions. The sequence and timing of the various treatments influence the likelihood of success. When we carefully listen to and watch the patient, he or she lets us know what interventions are needed, and when.

Effective treatment of chronic insomnia offers an exciting, pioneering realm of medical psychology. The psychological pain and life disruptiveness resulting from this condition are intense and widespread. A clear need exists for more professionals to provide urgently needed insomnia treatment. This comprehensive treatment model aims at breaking the vicious circle of insomnia and provides a method and structure to assist the clinician in delivering this greatly needed medical/psychological treatment.

Neil Steinberg is a licensed psychologist. For the seven years following receipt of his Ph.D. from California School of Professional Psychology, San Francisco, continued to provide psychiatric inpatient and outpatient services at Kaiser–Permanente Medical Center, Richmond City and Martinez City, California. In 1980 he created and began directing New Direction Adolescent Services, Inc., in Sonoma County, California, and in 1985 he began full-time private practice.

During 18 years of providing psychotherapeutic services, Dr. Steinberg has treated approximately 200 patients suffering from serious sleep loss. In 1987 he established Clinical Sleep Services in Sonoma County, California, to offer comprehensive insomnia treatment. Coordination with a sleep disorders neurologist and a local hospital-based polysomnography laboratory offers strong support for this urgently needed service.

RECOMMENDED READINGS

Coates, T. J., & Thoresen, C. E. (1977). *How to sleep better: A drug free program for overcoming insomnia.* Englewood Cliffs, NJ: Prentice-Hall.
  Behavioral management approaches for sleeplessness are presented clearly and thoroughly.
Kales, K., & Kales, J. (1984). *The evaluation and treatments of insomnia.* New York: Oxford University Press.
  A comprehensive overview with emphasis on psychotherapeutic interventions for insomnia.
Mason, L. J. (1985). *Guide to stress reduction.* Berkeley, CA: Celestial Arts Publishers.
  The mind–body relaxation techniques applied to insomnia treatment are fully discussed and described.

REFERENCES

Ascher, L. M., & Turner, R. M. (1978). Paradoxical intention and insomnia: An experimental investigation. In *Proceedings of the International Congress of Behavioral Therapy.* Vienna, Austria: International Congress of Behavioral Therapy.
Bootzin, R. R., & Nicassio, P. M. (1978). Behavioral treatments from insomnia. *Progress in Behavior Modification, 6,* 1–45.
Evans, D., & Bond, I. (1969). Reciprocal inhibition therapy and classical conditioning in the treatment of insomnia. *Behavioral Research and Therapy, 7,* 323–325.
Frankl, V. (1960). Paradoxical intention. *American Journal of Psychotherapy, 14,* 520-535.
Hauri, P. J. (1982). The sleep disorders. In *Current concepts, a scope publication.* Kalamazoo, MI: The Upjohn Company.

Hauri, P. J., Percy, L., Hellekson, C., Hartmann, E., & Luss, D. (1982). The treatment of psychophysiologic insomnia with biofeedback: A replication study. *Biofeedback Self Regulation, 7,* 223–235.

Haynes, S. N., Price, M. G., & Simons, J. B. (1975). Stimulus control treatment of insomnia. *Journal of Behavioral Therapy and Experimental Psychiatry, 6,* 279–282.

Jacobson, E. (1983). *Progressive relaxation.* Chicago: University of Chicago Press.

Kales, K., & Kales, J. (1984). *The evaluation and treatments of insomnia.* New York: Oxford University Press.

Lazarus, A. A. (1976). *Multimodal behavior therapy.* New York: Springer.

Ribordy, S. C., & Denney, D. R. (1977). The behavioral treatment of insomnia, an alternative to drug therapy. *Behavioral Research Therapy, 15,* 39–50.

Soldatos, C. R., Kales, A., & Kales, J. (1979). Management of insomnia. *Annual Review of Medicine, 30,* 301–312.

Spielman, A., Saskin, P., & Thorpy, M. (1987). Treatment of chronic insomnia by restriction of time in bed. *Sleep, 10*(1), 45–56.

Thoresen, C. E., Coates, T. J., Kirmil-Gray, K., & Rosekind, M. R. (1981). Behavioral self-management in treating sleep maintenance insomnia. *Journal of Behavioral Medicine, 4,* 41–52.

Turner, R. M., & Ascher, L. M. (1979). Controlled comparison of progressive relaxation, stimulus control and paradoxical intention therapies for insomnia. *Journal of Consulting and Clinical Psychology, 47,* 500–508.

Woolfolk, R. L., Carr-Kaffashan, L., McNulty, T. F., & Lehrer, P. M. (1976). Meditation training as a treatment for insomnia. *Behavioral Therapy, 7,* 359–365.

CHAPTER ELEVEN

Sleep Behavior Management

SIDNEY D. NAU, JOHN H. KOEWLER, AND JAMES K. WALSH

INTRODUCTION

We have used an educationally oriented treatment program termed "sleep behavior management" (SBM) in the treatment of insomnia. The program emphasizes factors known to influence sleep and their integration into an individual's life-style. SBM is a structured treatment, with active patient involvement and carefully selected behaviors. The basic premise of SBM is the interdependence of sleep and waking behaviors. Although sleep cannot be directly controlled, substantial influence over it can be obtained by manipulating waking behavior. Patients are taught to systematically implement sleep behavior principles to improve sleep quality and quantity. At the end of therapy, independent management of sleep behavior is possible and expected.

SBM assumes a multidetermined nature for sleep disturbance and presenting complaints. Treatment incorporates a variety of biological, psychological, and social factors that researchers have shown influence sleep. The often demonstrated fact that patient–therapist relationship plays a crucial role in treatment outcome is also emphasized. The focus of treatment is promotion of behaviors that favor sleep and elimination of obstacles to sleep. The general treatment scheme involves a structured hypothesis-testing process to organize and monitor sleep behavior changes. The process resembles a series of single patient treatment trials with continuous monitoring of results.

Sidney D. Nau, John H. Koewler, and James K. Walsh • Sleep Disorders and Research Center, Deaconess Hospital, St. Louis, Missouri 63139.

PATIENT SELECTION AND MANAGEMENT

Routine diagnostic evaluation includes a thorough history and physical, psychological evaluation, and, in some cases, polysomnography. This process excludes patients with primary diagnoses best addressed with medical or psychiatric treatment (e.g., sleep apnea, psychiatric disorder, drug dependency insomnia). Such patients may be candidates for the outlined treatment as an adjunct to their primary therapy or after resolution of the primary disorder.

It is the norm that patient distress and the need for change are not nearly enough to energize positive behavior changes in response to therapeutic recommendations. In some cases, patients have extreme difficulty concentrating on instructions and accepting prescribed intervention because most of their energy is expended on maladaptive coping strategies. Such individuals are most likely to comply with recommended behavioral changes when they also receive supportive psychotherapy. Also, the anxiety, frustration, confusion, and depressed mood that often accompany insomnia interfere with treatment compliance if they are not addressed. Supportive psychotherapy involves encouragement, understanding, clarification of behavioral and emotional problems, and confrontation when necessary.

On the other hand, many insomnia patients do not need psychotherapy. Their frustration and anxiety are more sleep-specific, less global, and tend to occur in the sleep setting. In our experience, relaxation training or cognitive restructuring is an effective first step in the systematic behavioral approach.

GENERAL TREATMENT SCHEME

Just as important as the specific behaviors needing change are the more general principles and strategies that patients are instructed to use to guide their behavior change efforts. As already noted, SBM is an educational/learning–based approach. The training follows behavior therapy principles such as individualized functional analysis* of symptoms

---

*Within a behavioral model, the therapist's first job is defining problem behavior (dependent variable; e.g., wakefulness during the sleep period) and the factors maintaining that behavior (independent variable; e.g., nocturnal overarousal, negative conditioning). In other words, the therapist as an empirical scientist attempts to develop with the patient a clear definition of the presenting problem and its causes. This is referred to as the "functional analysis of behavior", although the more traditional label of "assessment" or the term "behavioral assessment" may also be used (Craighead, Kazdin, & Mahoney, 1981).

and causes and continuous assessment during treatment (e.g., daily sleep logs). Sleep logs result in feedback which permits continuous development of the individualized treatment plan. Each treatment step is thus subject to data-based validation and is a small-scale monitored treatment trial. These behavior therapy principles are taught to clients as a multistep hypothesis-testing approach. Within this approach, each stage in treatment follows a three-step process consisting of (1) identification of sleep-related behaviors in need of change, (2) selection of one or two sleep behavior changes most likely to have positive impact on sleep, (3) initiation of a treatment trial period with collection of daily sleep–wake pattern data via sleep logs. Selection of new behavior changes sometimes occurs at every visit. The patient is instructed to alter his/her pattern of sleep behaviors gradually in order to have realistic, achievable goals, to avoid undue stress, and to facilitate assessment of efficacy. Assessment of effectiveness is critical. It allows the patient to know what changes significantly decreased symptomatology. After each trial period the three-step cycle is repeated: (1) reassessment of patient sleep status to judge the results of treatment, (2) formulation of the next stage of treatment, e.g., revise previously implemented changes, add new changes, (3) initiation of the next trial period to test newly formulated steps in the treatment process. At termination, successful intervention is reviewed and the patient is instructed to use this knowledge in the future if sleep quality deteriorates.

An integral aspect of the self-management philosophy of SBM is the use of questionnaires and educational handouts. Information is reviewed with the patient at each visit and copies are sent home with her/him. Questionnaires are used for pre-, and post-, and ongoing treatment assessments. These include a brief daily sleep log, a log for behavior change goals, and instructional handouts that describe treatment components (to facilitate ease and accuracy of home practice).

IMPLEMENTATION OF SLEEP BEHAVIOR MANAGEMENT

The initial session has two major components: (1) education and (2) treatment planning.

Patient education is begun during session 1. Much of the material covered falls under the general rubric of "sleep hygiene" (Zarcone, 1989). That is, patients are given instruction on the effects of caffeine, alcohol, and other drugs, the importance of a regular sleep–wake schedule (particularly morning wakeup time), the deleterious effects of naps (rarely, the desirability of naps), the need for a presleep routine, and so forth. Additionally, patients acquire a fundamental knowledge base to allow them to be active participants in treatment decisions and to help them after completion of treatment. For example, basic information is presented on interindividual variability in sleep need, sleep deprivation effects, circadian rhythms, and daily stress effects on sleep. Although the sleep environment needs to be comfortable, patients learn that occasional awakenings due to neighborhood noise, light in the room, and the like are usually not fundamental to insomnia. Emphasis is placed on the fact that many things that improve sleep are under their control. In fact, convincing patients that the quality and/or quantity of sleep is often under their direct or indirect control may be more important than the actual information presented. That is, waking behaviors markedly influence sleep (and vice versa) and regaining "control" over sleep often requires extreme regulation of waking behaviors, at least temporarily. Patient resistance to this principle is a frequent early sign that psychotherapy, at some level, is likely to be needed. It may signal a "passive victim" view of illness or that secondary gain is considerable. Certainly it guides the therapist in formation of the patient–therapist relationship.

Treatment planning focuses on further delineation of specific etiological factors and assignment of relative importance to each, not necessarily with regard to the onset or development of the sleep disturbance, but rather the relative importance with regard to initiating successful intervention. Three general concerns are probed and examined in more detail: current sleep status, past efforts to improve sleep, and perceived causes for the patient's complaints (see Table 1).

Initial behavior goals are chosen based on patient assessment, yet some goals are so frequently selected they are dominant in therapist efforts to help the new patient. The following are examples of initial behavior goals that have had proven value in generating patient expectancy of relief and, in turn, therapist feelings of competency. Thus, they can foster early encouragement for patient and therapist. Relaxation training is often an initial goal and is discussed at length below as a model goal. Efforts to foster positive conditioning experiences (Bootzin, 1972) are basic to full resolution of most insomnia problems and sometimes represent goal 1. A cognitive restructuring approach might begin by articulating and attacking problem attitudes that underlie the patient's perspective on insomnia; e.g., insomnia is incapacitating, the ability to sleep has been lost or drastically altered, the problem is so chronic that it is hopeless, or other irrational beliefs. At times, pharmacotherapy has a role in SBM. The early use of hypnotic medications often provides relief from acute distress and allows greater readiness for more analytical and behavioral steps. Other possible initial goals include direct manipulations of worry behavior (e.g., with prescription of special times and places for worry) and discontinua-

Table 1. Patient Assessment Topics

I. Details of current sleep management
   a. Sleep schedule
   b. Analysis of activities during the one to two hours before bedtime
   c. Bedtime routine
   d. Emotional and behavioral responses to long periods of wakefulness during the sleep period
   e. Analysis of the bedroom environment
   f. Social factors related to insomnia, e.g., sleep disturbance by the bed partner, negative effects of insomnia behavior on the spouse
   g. Sleep needs
   h. Amount of experience with relaxation training
   i. Evidence for conditioning as a causal factor
   j. Negative thought processes, e.g., exaggerated fear of insomnia
   k. Intake of caffeine, nicotine, and other substances that affect sleep and/or alertness

II. Past efforts to improve sleep
   a. Cognitive techniques, e.g., concentration on one thing (e.g., counting sheep), prayer, cognitive relaxation training, self-hypnosis
   b. Sleep-promoting medication or alcohol
   c. Somatic treatment (e.g., pain medication, chiropractic, endocrine therapy, dietary changes)
   d. Other techniques, e.g., listening to music, exercise, muscle relaxation training, relaxing imagery

III. Patient's perceived causes for insomnia
   a. Excessive cognitive activity, e.g., planning future activities, reviewing the day, reminiscing, and, often, worrying about sleep
   b. Physiological overarousal
   c. Poor sleep hygiene
   d. Sleep-disturbing environmental stimuli
   e. Iatrogenic factors
   f. Organic disorder

tion of hypnotic medications. These initial behavior change goals are offered as examples; the clinician must limit the number of initial goals to one or two at the first session.

Continuous self-assessment of sleep–wake status through sleep logs is necessary, particularly early in treatment. This is taught during session 1.

Cognitive (meditative) relaxation is often taught during session 1, particularly with patients who perceive overarousal to be contributing to insomnia. Relaxation training is provided as a behavioral method for decreasing arousal (Borkovec & Weerts, 1976) and as demonstration that individuals have the ability to influence somatic and mental activity which they may have felt was previously unachievable. It is a skill that improves with practice; thus early training facilitates early rewards. Most patients obtain some degree of immediate relaxation, i.e., during the first practice session. When the dearousing effects of relaxation can be felt, patient feelings of being out of control often decrease. Persistent insomnia almost always evokes strong perceptions of loss of control. Therefore, early and continuous efforts to build feelings of mastery are basic to treatment success.

We use cognitive relaxation strategies first [e.g., the meditative technique of Benson (1975)] because more patients report cognitive arousal than physiological arousal and the technique can be rapidly learned. Some patients succeed only with muscle relaxation techniques (Jacobsen, 1938), which are much more time-consuming, while others do best with visual imagery relaxation. It is desirable for each patient to receive a trial with different methods of relaxing.

At the end of session 1, the patient will typically have one or two behavior change goals (e.g., practice with relaxation procedures, begin hypnotic withdrawal, practice stimulus control) and will begin logging sleep–wake pattern.

Following session 1, remaining sessions address the following: (1) assessment of previous behavior change, (2) problem solving on more effective implementation of behavior change (as needed), (3) guidance in selection of behaviors to be altered during the next treatment period, (4) further instruction in relaxation techniques, (5) continuing education regarding pertinent sleep principles, and (6) supportive or ventilative psychotherapy, as necessary. The usual number of sessions ranges from four to eight.

During each session, a significant amount of time is devoted to instruction and guided practice in the process of empirical hypothesis testing. The patient is encouraged to formulate answers to the key questions of what behaviors need to be changed and what effects follow changes that are made. There is one week, minimum, between visits to facilitate evaluation of habit changes chosen at each session.

CASE STUDY (SUCCESSFUL)

Ms. K was a 32-year-old, single female referred by her physician for evaluation of sleep maintenance insomnia of three months' duration. The insomnia first occurred approximately two nights a week. Subsequently, the problem gradually increased until it had become a nightly problem for the last month.

The patient described a fairly consistent pattern of going to bed at 10:30 P.M., falling asleep quickly, then waking about 2:00 A.M., feeling "wide awake," and remaining awake for two to three hours, sometimes for the remainder of the night. Ms. K often had thoughts on her mind when awakening during the night and frequently was thinking of a tune which she could not dismiss. She denied excessive muscle tension at these times. The patient estimated she got three to six hours of sleep each night, getting up between 6:00 and 9:00 A.M. She had tried a number of things to improve her sleep, including getting out of bed to read, watch television, play the piano, paint, or clean house. None of these seemed to help. She had tried triazolam and an over-the-counter medication for several nights without benefit a few weeks prior to our evaluation. There was no history of medical illness, sleep apnea, or nocturnal myoclonus. No caffeine or alcohol abuse was indicated. A physical examination showed she was in good health.

The patient was very concerned that the insomnia was interfering with her life. She worked full time in the computer field and performed as an actress and singer in the evenings and on weekends. She was quite anxious that lack of adequate sleep would interfere with her acting, feeling that she needed to be "100 percent" to perform effectively. Although there was no clear evidence that her performance had suffered, she felt she was not doing her best and feared making a fool of herself on stage.

Conflict with her boyfriend appeared to be causing distress. There was a long-standing problem about the long-term stability of the relationship. She admitted to feelings of depression, which she insisted were a consequence of lack of sleep.

Preliminary diagnosis was insomnia associated with dysthymia with a possible psychophysiological component. Treatment was begun with administration of a low dose (25 mg) of amitriptyline, principally because of the sense of urgency expressed by the patient. An antidepressant was used because of the recent ineffectiveness of a benzodiazepine reported by the patient. Basic sleep hygiene instructions were also provided. Ms. K's insomnia improved promptly and dramatically. She continued to awaken one or two times a night, but she had no prolonged awakenings. We did not interpret this response as an antidepressant effect as the dose of amitriptyline was low and improvement occurred within a few days.

Psychological assessment indicated no serious depression but mild hysterical features. The patient appeared to have a strong need to be in control and typically repressed her emotional problems. Her perception of generally poor functioning and inability to control her sleep frightened her and contributed to the insomnia. It appeared she had an adjustment disorder with depressed mood, having reacted intensely to the insomnia and her perception of its effects on her. The relationship conflict was also deemed to be a significant stressor, perhaps contributing to the insomnia.

After one month, the patient agreed to discontinue the amitriptyline and begin SBM. The patient was seen in five biweekly appointments after the antidepressant had been discontinued. Initial behavior changes included maintaining a regular wakeup time and stimulus control procedures (see Chapter 2). Supportive psychotherapy before and during behavior change was instrumental in helping the patient feel less distressed about the insomnia. Empathy was expressed for her anxiety related to lack of control over sleep and the feared deterioration of life quality. The patient's interpersonal problems were also discussed, not in great depth, but enough to help her see their relevance as a stressor that needed to be addressed. This lessened her repression of the problems, enabling her to realize the need for conscious decisions about her relationships and social life.

During the first two weeks postmedication, daily logs indicated a pattern of sleeping well for several nights, then having three or four nights of sleep maintenance difficulty, much like her presenting complaint, then a return of good sleep. Ms. K quickly learned the value of making hypotheses regarding the contributing factors of her insomnia and the evaluation of behavior change strategies. An effective therapeutic alliance was established in which she felt like a responsible partner in the treatment of her problem. The most difficult problem she noted was that she felt "wide awake" when she was unable to return to sleep during the night. The patient observed that if she engaged in an enjoyable activity during the night, such as playing the piano or painting, she did not become drowsy, apparently because she enjoyed these activities and had inadequate time for them during the day. She was advised to read or watch television, which were less interesting, and which seemed to promote drowsiness.

Ms. K firmly adhered to her regular rising time and, when necessary, engaged in a monotonous activity during nighttime awakenings. Just as important, the patient began to recognize the interaction of stress in interpersonal relationships with sleep quality. Ambiguity in relationships was identified as very unsettling and anxiety producing, and therefore, goals were established to reduce this ambiguity, with positive results. Ms. K also benefitted from the knowledge that the degree of sleep loss she was experiencing was unlikely to significantly impair her acting ability. She felt less anxious and relieved in general, and performance anxiety (when attempting to sleep) was substantially reduced. Daily logs indicated that sleep maintenance difficulty gradually diminished during the next two months.

After five sessions, the patient reported that sleep maintenance was a problem only one night per week on the average. She was no longer anxious about the problem, feeling that she understood the insomnia better and had techniques to help reduce the problem when it occurred. A mutual decision to terminate SBM was made at that time.

Six weeks after her last visit, the patient returned because insomnia had recurred after a one-month period of nearly total remission. Ms. K reported essentially nightly sleep disturbance characterized by prolonged nocturnal awakenings, much like before. She was not nearly as distressed as during initial presentation, but decided to seek help again as the problem was persisting.

Previous behavior changes and treatment strategies were reviewed. Reevaluation indicated that her regular sleep–wake schedule had been maintained. No significant new stressors were noted. As before, the major problem appeared to be the patient's feeling of being "wide awake" when she awakened during the night. She reported having much creative energy which appeared to have insufficient outlet during the day. She often had "music playing" in her mind when she lay awake at night, and this was stimulating rather than relaxing for her. Even listening to music during awakenings seemed to be arousing rather than promoting drowsiness. On a few nights she enjoyed playing the piano or painting for hours during awakenings. The need to avoid stimulating activities at night was reviewed and clarified. The need to seek appropriate creative outlets during the day was determined. As before, reading at night helped her gradually feel drowsy, but returning to bed after she finished reading seemed to make her feel awake again. Because of this, the patient hypothesized that remaining in bed while reading would promote drowsiness, even though this was counter to the instruction. Based on the hypothesis-testing model, which can accommodate flexible behavior change strategies, the patient implemented this behavior change with positive results. Sleep logs indicated marked improvement over the subsequent two weeks. The improvement with this behavior change reduced the patient's anxiety about inability to control her return to sleep. Ms. K has continued to sleep well for the past six months, only rarely troubled by a long awakening.

CASE STUDY (UNSUCCESSFUL)

Mrs. C, an 83-year-old woman, was self-referred with a 13-year history of sleep-maintenance insomnia and hypnotic dependency. She and Mr. C, who urged her to seek help, were worried about her nightly use of flurazepam during the last three years. The patient reported one self-motivated effort to terminate medication, which was abruptly aborted due to nightmares. Hypnotic dependency had become a cause for self-criticism and fear of negative health consequences. At presentation, Mrs. C was taking 30 mg flurazepam to return to sleep after her second long awakening of the night.

During initial consultation, bedtime was reported to be regular at 9:30 P.M.; however, questionnaires later showed a more variable bedtime, ranging from 8:00 P.M. to 11:45 P.M. Sleep-onset latency averaged 10 to 20 minutes. Mrs. C reported frequent 30- to 60-minute awakenings during which she usually lay quietly in bed. During the second awakening, she would take flurazepam. As later awakenings were often accompanied by back pain, acetaminophen was often taken. Time of arising was between 6:30 and 7:30 A.M. There was no history of myoclonus, snoring, or observed apnea. It was her norm to take a 30- to 60-minute afternoon or early-evening nap. The absence of adequate evening activities for stimulation and/or pleasure was an irritation for Mrs. C. Thirteen years earlier Mrs. C had married her present husband, her second. When they married, she retired from secretarial work, moved from a city to a small, rural town, and adopted the relatively bland life-style of her husband. A weekly church group meeting was the only source of social stimulation. She described herself as a worrier. During nighttime awakenings and during the day, she worried about the consequences of poor sleep.

The patient claimed to be in good health with the exception of chronic back pain since age 16. She emphasized pain as a problem, but also claimed expertise in self-treatment. In addition to flurazepam and acetaminophen, medications taken were propranolol and hydrochlorothiazide for hypertension.

Due to the patient's age, the initial recommendation was polysomnography to screen for myoclonus or a sleep-related breathing abnormality. This was declined based on the belief that Mrs. C had a "pure" insomnia with hypnotic dependency and resistance to other interpretations. Therefore, SBM was begun.

Several negative behaviors were noted as potential obstacles to better sleep: hypnotic intake, daily napping, excessive worry, and back pain. More hypothetical factors were anxiety, anger, and frustration in the evening as a consequence of her unrewarding life-style.

Mrs. C approached the therapy situation with a talkative, vivacious, outgoing manner that suggested a high need for attention. The clinician gave close, sympathetic attention to her statements to increase the reward value of treatment sessions. She and her husband appeared highly motivated for hypnotic withdrawal and development of a new approach to sleep.

In session 1, assessment questionnaires were reviewed with the patient to further evaluate her perspective on insomnia. She suspected that something about her new life with Mr. C had caused her problem, as she had formerly been a good sleeper. Sleeping pills were the only treatment previously tried. Her main behavior change goal was discontinuation of hypnotic medication, yet she doubted her "body's ability" to sleep and thus feared permanent dependency on hypnotics. Her desired treatment outcome was decreased nighttime awakenings with increased daytime energy, and she was advised that until she had been sleeping for a few weeks without hypnotic intake, she should not expect to reestablish a more normal sleep–wake pattern. Patient education activities included sleep hygiene instruction and discussion of normative data for her age. Problematic sleep behaviors were noted as they were revealed during assessment of current sleep behaviors.

During a recent three-week vacation her symptoms had slackened, suggesting negative conditioning and the probable benefit of stimulus control procedures. In summary, the following negative behaviors were identified at the first session:

1. Chronic nightly use of hypnotic
2. Daily napping
3. Negative conditioning
4. Low level of social stimulation (relative to patient expectations)
5. Lack of relaxation in the evening
6. Excessive worry over sleep complaints
7. No experience with relaxation training
8. Chronic back pain complaints
9. Irregular bedtime routine

Initial behavior change goals were specified by the therapist and patient jointly:

1. Omit flurazepam one day in the next week and one additional day during each succeeding week.
2. Avoid daytime naps.
3. Complete daily sleep and activity logs.

It was also suggested that she try acetaminophen at bedtime to prevent need for an analgesic later in the night.

The patient returned 17 days later with the sleep logs, which indicated poor compliance. She omitted four flurazepam doses in 17 days. She continued to take one daily nap owing to persistent daytime tiredness. Mrs. C did not shift acetaminophen to bedtime, owing to her belief that maximal benefits would be obtained if the analgesic was taken close to her worst time for long awakenings.

The daily log showed no clear or consistent changes in reported sleep characteristics. One of her best nights of sleep was on a night without flurazepam. This was pointed out as evidence of the lack of total dependence on hypnotics.

Mrs. C was encouraged to discontinue napping on a trial basis, and she again agreed. She defended her continued napping by stating that unless she took her nap, she would be overly sleepy and nervous at bedtime. It was only on the day of her evening church group that the nap was omitted, without ill effects. Unsatisfying, inactive life-style was again suggested as a problem in her sleep–wake behavior pattern.

Mrs. C revealed that at night she worried a great deal about her heart racing. Therefore, cognitive relaxation was begun, to provide a way of decreasing arousal during awakenings. She became relaxed and drowsy during a 10- to 15-minute training session and was enthusiastic afterward.

Two additional goals were specified at the end of session 2:

1. Daily home relaxation practice, particularly at bedtime and at the beginning of awakenings.
2. Follow the most basic rule of stimulus control treatment: "the bed is for sleep." She was instructed to get out of bed after 30 minutes of wakefulness, to engage in a quiet, relaxing activity.

On the thirty-eighth day of treatment, the patient returned for session 3. Mrs. C's *last* flurazepam tablet had been taken four days earlier and naps were omitted on an intermittent basis, without apparent ill effect. She had followed the 30-minute rule only once or twice during three weeks.

Mrs. C's sleep remained consistent throughout the withdrawal process. She had occasional mild to moderate delay in sleep onset, several long awakenings each night, and a nightly early final awakening. Her stable sleep pattern was again discussed as evidence of success and limited need for sleep medication.

Nausea and abdominal discomfort had increased during the later weeks of flurazepam withdrawal. A new physician she consulted offered chlordiazepoxide, but she declined due to fear of dependency. Low back pain increased, for which she began taking ibuprofen.

We discussed what to do when she got out of bed during long awakenings. Radio was suggested as an eyes-open activity for times when she got up. She had rejected reading, watching television, or handwork owing to her poor vision. Mrs. C expressed significant hesitancy to get up for fear of disturbing her husband, but again accepted it as a goal.

Behavior change goals added during session 3 included the following:

1. Mrs. C decided to seek more frequent daytime and evening social occasions, as this was relaxing and helped decrease napping.
2. In a continuing effort to institute stimulus control procedures, she was to identify a few solitary and relaxing nighttime activities for use in management of long awakenings.

Session 4 occurred 21 days after session 3 and two months after the beginning of treatment. Mrs. C had taken no flurazepam for three weeks. The sleep pattern remained stable, with consistent complaints of excessive daytime sleepiness. She failed again to consistently omit naps, but no negative outcome was noted when naps were omitted. She remained noncompliant with the 30-minute rule. Mrs. C continued to emphasize physical complaints, reporting more stomach upset and increasing back pain, plus agitation. She had become so upset on one occasion that Mr. C took her to an emergency room, where evaluation was negative.

Owing to Mrs. C's low compliance, increased somatic complaints, and emotionality, she was asked to complete the Minnesota Multiphasic Personality Inventory (MMPI) during session 4. The results showed a strong tendency to develop somatic complaints in reaction to psychological problems, associated risk for secondary gain, and possible depression.

No new behavior change goals were set, to avoid new stressors. Prior goals were reviewed. In an effort to provide emotional support, the therapist directed Mrs. C to call after her bad nights.

The fourth training session was Mrs. C's last. She rescheduled the next visit three times, twice due to back pain and once because of her husband's illness. She called once after a bad night and reported that such special contact did help her worry less and cope better. After canceling her visit for the third time, Mrs. C suspended treatment indefinitely, in part due to uncertainty about insurance. The insurer eventually paid her bill, but she has not returned despite complimentary remarks on the helpfulness of therapy.

This patient's treatment was impressive for its success with gradual withdrawal from chronic hypnotic use in an older individual. Other treatment interventions that may have enhanced successful treatment include the following:

1. Mrs. C was willing to give up sleeping pills, but slow to try new behaviors. The therapist should have aggressively adjusted for this patient's resistance to change, e.g., by programming smaller behavior change steps. He/she should have been ready to change goals after noncompliance. Psychotherapeutic analysis of resistance might have been helpful. In other words, patient inflexibility calls for very high therapist innovation. As another example, a more active role for the patient's husband might have provided needed support at home.
2. Perhaps pain was a significant factor and the patient would have benefitted from direct treatment with an analgesic.
3. Mrs. C's lack of enjoyment and stimulation may have produced

significant anxiety, which had previously been attenuated by flurazepam, a long-acting compound. This possible benefit of carry-over sedation was not explained to Mrs. C, and the potential problems caused by loss of daytime sedation were not addressed.
4. Mrs. C was oriented toward medical/somatic analysis of insomnia. Her belief in the medical risks of chronic hypnotic use was a prime motivator that aided withdrawal from sleeping pills. However, she was given no medically/somatically oriented substitute.
5. Mrs C's heavy focus on somatic complaints and resistance to behavior change were consistent with her MMPI results. Successful psychotherapeutic intervention for a somatization tendency might have improved compliance.
6. Mrs. C's agitation and helplessness near the end of treatment had the flavor of agitated depression. She might have benefitted from antidepressant medication and/or psychotherapy.
7. It would be highly desirable to perform a polysomnographic evaluation, which might reveal occult causes for Mrs. C's stalemate in treatment.

Sidney D. Nau received a Ph.D. in Clinical Psychology from the University of Iowa in 1977. His work with sleep disorders began in 1972 as a team member in some of the earliest efforts to demonstrate behavior therapy's applicability to insomnia. He was a postdoctoral fellow at the Deaconess Hospital Sleep Disorders and Research Center in St. Louis (1982–1984) and returned there in 1989 after developing an independent sleep disorders center elsewhere in St. Louis. Dr. Nau is a fellow of the American Sleep Disorders Association.

John H. Koewler received a Ph.D in Clinical Psychology from the University of Miami. He served as staff clinical psychologist at the Deaconess Hospital Sleep Disorders and Research Center for three years during which time he specialized in behavioral and psychological intervention for insomnia. Since 1989, he has been in private practice in St. Louis.

James K. Walsh received a Ph.D. in Experimental Psychology from St. Louis University in 1976. He has been active in sleep research since 1974 and in 1981 founded the Sleep Disorders and Research Center at Deaconess Hospital in St. Louis. He is also Associate Clinical Professor in the Departments of Psychiatry, Neurology, and Pediatrics at the St. Louis University School of Medicine. Dr. Walsh has served on the board of directors of the American Sleep Disorders Association since 1984 and is currently President-elect.

RECOMMENDED READINGS

Coates, T. J., & Thoresen, C. E. (1977). *How to sleep better: A drug-free program for overcoming insomnia.* Englewood Cliffs, NJ: Prentice-Hall.
A patient-oriented manual for self-management of insomnia.

Lacks, P. (1987). *Behavioral treatment for persistent insomnia.* New York: Pergamon Press.
A recent manual of behavior therapy techniques for insomnia designed for the practitioner.

Spielman, A. J. (1986). Assessment of insomnia. *Clinical Psychology Review, 6,* 11–25.
A review of behavioral assessment for insomnia with interesting theoretical comments.

Spielman, A. J., Caruso, L. S., & Glovinsky, P. B. (1987). A behavioral perspective on insomnia treatment. *Psychiatric Clinics of North America, 10,* 541–553.
A discussion of the behavioral point of view and behavior therapies for insomnia.

REFERENCES

Benson, H. (1975). *The relaxation response.* New York: Morrow.

Bootzin, R. R. (1972). Stimulus control treatment for insomnia (Summary). *Proceedings of the 80th Annual Convention of the American Psychological Association, 1,* 395–396.

Borkovec, T. D., & Weerts, T. C. (1976). Effects of progressive relaxation on sleep disturbance: An electroencephalographic evaluation. *Psychosomatic Medicine, 38,* 173–180.

Craighead, W. E., Kazdin, A. E., & Mahoney, M. J. (1981). *Behavior modification: Principles, issues and applications* (2nd ed.). Boston: Houghton Mifflin, pp 159–160.

Jacobsen, E. (1938). *Progressive relaxation.* Chicago: University of Chicago Press.

Zarcone, V. P. (1989). Sleep hygiene. In M. H. Kryger, T. Roth, & W. C. Dement (Eds.), *Principles and practice of sleep medicine.* Philadelphia: W. B. Saunders Co.

Part Four

Disorders of the Sleep–Wake Schedule

Not all insomnia is the result of emotional turmoil and inappropriate behaviors. Misalignment of the circadian rhythm may be a major cause of insomnia. Part Four deals with that aspect. In Chapter Twelve, Russell Rosenberg discusses the treatment of delayed sleep phase syndromes, i.e., the treatment of patients who have great difficulty falling asleep before the early morning hours and then sleep quite well until noon, or later. The bright-light therapy he describes is an exciting new addition to the armamentarium of insomnia therapists. Being able to reset the hands of the circadian clock by light makes it possible to change sleep to the appropriate hours. Chronotherapy, i.e., the delaying of sleep by three to four hours each night until one goes to bed around 10 or 11 P.M., is a somewhat older, but still efficient, method to achieve the same goal. However, as Rosenberg justly points out, there may be complicating factors, such as substance abuse and a socially reinforced delayed sleep phase, which make the treatment of delayed sleep phase syndromes more complex than meets the eye.

In Chapter Thirteen, Richard Allen deals with the opposite: early morning awakenings. Typically, this symptom used to be interpreted as indicating endogenous depression, but Allen shows that many cases of early morning awakenings can be treated by exposure to bright light in the evening, while avoiding light in the morning. This schedule of light treatment delays sleep onset in the evening and increases sleepiness during the early morning hours.

CHAPTER TWELVE

Assessment and Treatment of Delayed Sleep Phase Syndrome

RUSSELL ROSENBERG

INTRODUCTION

Delayed sleep phase syndrome can be a very frustrating and debilitating problem for patients. It often results in poor school or work histories, family discord, disturbed social relationships, and, at times, depression related to the intractable and uncontrollable nature of the disorder. This sleep–wake schedule disorder is characterized by a chronic inability to sleep at a desired or "socially acceptable" hour. Sleep onset is often delayed until early morning (3:00 to 6:00 A.M.) with a usual arousal time of late morning to early afternoon (11:00 A.M. to 3:00 P.M.). Otherwise, sleep is "normal." A history of being a "night owl" is typical. Over an extended time period, the cumulative sleep debt often leads patients to complain of daytime somnolence. In an effort to cope with the disorder, patients may self-medicate with hypnotics or alcohol to help them get to sleep and with stimulants to decrease daytime sleepiness. Therefore, a substance abuse problem may also complicate the diagnosis and subsequent treatment.

Insomnia due to delayed sleep phase syndrome presents a significant clinical challenge. Over the years, I have found delayed sleep phase syndrome to be one of the most misunderstood and overlooked causes of insomnia.

Russell Rosenberg • Northside Hospital, Atlanta, Georgia 30342.

BACKGROUND

The prevalence and incidence of delayed sleep phase syndrome have not yet been determined. This disorder may be the most common problem of the sleep–wake schedule in patients seen at sleep disorders centers (Coleman, Roffwarg, Kennedy, Guilleminault, Cinque, Cohn, Karacan, Kupfer, Lemmi, Miles, Orr, Phillips, Roth, Sassin, Schmidt, & Dement, 1982). In the national cooperative study, Coleman *et al.* (1982) found that approximately 40 percent of patients with a disorder of the sleep–wake schedule were diagnosed with delayed sleep phase syndrome. Unfortunately, an accurate estimate of the prevalence of delayed sleep phase syndrome cannot be obtained from this cooperative study.

It has been suggested that delayed sleep phase patients present at a younger age than the average insomnia patient (Weitzman, Czeisler, Coleman, Spielman, Zimmerman, & Dement, 1981). Pelayo, Thorpy, and Glovinsky (1988) examined the prevalence of delayed sleep phase syndrome in a group of adolescents. They found that the disorder is relatively common in this population. Approximately 7 percent of their sample reported having symptoms suggestive of delayed sleep phase syndrome on their questionnaires. It is evident that a randomized, national survey is needed to determine the incidence and prevalence of delayed sleep phase syndrome in both children and adults.

Basic principles and properties of the endogenous circadian pacemaker are important to consider when making a diagnosis or developing a treatment plan. These properties include: its intrinsic cycle length, stable position during entrainment, amplitude of oscillation, and resetting capacity. In a "free running" period, the human circadian cycle averages about 25 hours (Wever, 1979). However, recent evidence suggests that a circadian rhythm significantly longer than 24 hours may be found mainly in adolescents and young adults (e.g., 15 to 30 years old). While the data supporting this notion are sparse, they may explain why the majority of delayed sleep phase syndrome patients present at an earlier age than other insomniacs. On a daily basis, the endogenous pacemaker resets itself by exposure to a number of environmental stimuli (light–dark, social cues).

Attempts to understand the pathophysiology of delayed sleep phase syndrome have been made by examining the phase-response curve demonstrated in plants and animals. The phase-response curve is a mathematical representation of an organism's likelihood for changing its circadian cycle. Essentially it is used to determine whether nonentrained subjects can be entrained by stimuli presented at various times on the curve. In a delayed sleep phase syndrome patient, the range of entrainment may be quite narrow and limited. Most people have much greater difficulty shortening their days (e.g., to 22 hours) than they have lengthening their days (e.g., to 26 hours), probably because the innate biological rhythm typically is 25 hours. While the mechanism of the phase response curve is not fully understood, the result for delayed sleep phase patients is an inability to phase-advance each day, with a delayed phase becoming the consistent sleep pattern.

A relationship between psychiatric illness and delayed sleep phase syndrome has not been empirically established. Weitzman *et al.* (1981) found the two to be unrelated and suggested that psychiatric-type symptoms (cognitive rumination) were a consequence of the disorder. Mendelson (1987) suggested that there may be a relationship between psychiatric illness and delayed sleep phase syndrome. He reported that many, if not most, of his patients with this disorder have histories of depression or character disorder. I have also found evidence of psychopathology in this group of patients [Minnesota Multiphasic Personality Inventory (MMPI) clinical scales above 70] and agree with Mendelson's recommendation that the issue be considered unsettled until further case series have been conducted.

Treatments for the delayed sleep phase syndrome have been developed in consideration of its pathophysiology. Czeisler, Richardson, Coleman, Zimmerman, Moore-Ede, Dement, and Weitzman (1981) proposed treating delayed sleep phase patients with chronotherapy. Chronotherapy is a behavioral treatment during which the patient is instructed to go to bed three hours later each night, essentially establishing a 27-hour activity–rest cycle. The patient continues to delay the sleep–wake schedule around the clock until the desired bedtime is reached. At that point, a 24-hour schedule is enforced by having the patient maintain a regular arousal time. Czeisler *et al.* (1981) based their treatment on the knowledge that the endogenous circadian cycle is longer than 24 hours, therefore making it easier to delay the sleep–wake cycle rather than advancing it. In their study, five patients underwent successful chronotherapy.

Ceizler *et al.* (1981) emphasized that once the patient achieves the desired schedule, he/she needs to rigorously maintain it by not varying the sleep–wake cycle. The sleep–wake schedule of these patients are very fragile, and they must be made aware of the consequences of returning to a delayed schedule for even one night! Chronotherapy has been successfully used in time isolation facilities and in the home environment. However, few time isolation facilities exist and the expense to the patient can be prohibitive. Difficulties with family cooperation and patient compliance can arise when treatment is conducted at home, and these problems must be anticipated and discussed with the patient.

Early morning exercise may also be a potential treatment for delayed sleep phase syndrome patients. Piercy and Lack (1988) found that intense aerobic exercise in the morning, independent of light exposure, has phase-advancing potential.

Lewy, Singer, and Sack (1985) found that exposure to bright light can shift the circadian rhythm of core body temperature and rapid-eye-movement propensity. Their conclusion was that the delayed sleep phase syndrome can be treated by scheduling successively earlier wake times with one to two hours of bright-light exposure immediately after waking up.

Vanderpool, Rosenthal, Levendosky, Johnston, Allen, Kelly, Soutre, Schultz, and Stafz (1989) also reported successfully treating delayed sleep phase syndrome patients with bright light. The diagnosis of delayed sleep phase syndrome was based on interviews, one month of sleep diary data, wrist activity monitors which measured motion and were used to predict sleep periods, and polysomnographic studies. Patients were randomly assigned to one of two groups. One group received exposure of 2500 lux full-spectrum light for two hours in the morning between 6:00 A.M. and 9:00 A.M. and wore dark goggles in the late afternoon, 4:00 P.M. to dusk. The other group was exposed to 300 lux at the same time and wore clear goggles in the late afternoon to dusk. Results indicated that a phase advance took place in the group exposed to 2500 lux but not in the control group. The authors concluded that bright light presented on awakening can advance the circadian rhythms of delayed sleep phase syndrome patients.

Despite the suggestion that pharmacological treatments alone are ineffective (Weitzman *et al.*, 1981), Uruha, Mikami, Teshima, Sugita, Honda, Inatani, Taehibana, Egawa, Tsutsumi, and Iijima (1987) reported successfully treating two delayed sleep phase syndrome patients with triazolam. They administered 0.25 mg (case 1) and a hefty 0.5 mg (case 2) of triazolam at a time when the patient was still awake but wanted to be sleeping (two to four hours before desired bedtime). These authors concluded that triazolam can be an effective treatment for delayed sleep phase syndrome. Vanderpool, Kelly, Schultz, Allen, Souetre, and Rosenthal (1988) suggested that a combination of triazolam and bright light be considered for treating delayed sleep phase syndrome patients. They reported anecdotally that one of their patients noted an improved ability to comply with the light treatment when given triazolam to take whenever problems initiating sleep arose. While a combined treatment approach is appealing, additional studies are needed to determine whether triazolam or other medications can aid in the treatment of delayed sleep phase syndrome.

METHOD

The complex multidimensional nature of insomnia demands a comprehensive, multimethod approach. This is especially true for making the diagnosis of delayed sleep phase syndrome. At our sleep disorders center, we utilize: sleep history questionnaires, observer data (bed partner questionnaire and interview when available), clinical interview, psychological tests such as the MMPI and Beck Depression Inventory, medical evaluation, and polysomnography. When patients are referred to the Sleep Disorders Center, they usually have a two- to three-week wait for the initial evaluation. They are sent a packet of information, sleep history questionnaire, and a two-week sleep diary to complete prior to their appointment. Patients are told to expect to spend about three hours at the Sleep Disorders Center for the initial assessment.

Upon arrival at the Center, each patient undergoes a brief orientation and is instructed to complete the MMPI. After completion, a 60- to 90-minute clinical interview is conducted. The sleep history questionnaire is reviewed and discussed with the patient. Medical history is also reviewed. If the patient has not had a physical examination including blood laboratory evaluation (e.g., complete blood count, sedimentation rate, SMA 18, and thyroid profile) in the past three months, an evaluation is conducted and the appropriate laboratory studies are carried out. If there has been a recent examination, we request these records for our review. A drug screen is also conducted at the time of the initial evaluation to assess for potential drug use which may affect the sleep–wake cycle (e.g., stimulants and depressants). This is our basic intake protocol regardless of presenting complaint.

If a persistent delayed sleep pattern emerges from the intake data, and the delayed sleep phase is not due to use of stimulants or other medications that might inhibit sleep onset at "normal" hours, laboratory polysomnography is conducted for two nights. We utilize standard polysomnographic techniques and scoring procedures. On night 1 we begin the study at the time the patient usually attempts sleep, say at 11:00 P.M., and allow sleep to continue approximately to the usual wakeup time. On night 2, the study begins at the time of the "normal" sleep tendency, say at 3:00 A.M. This information is obtained from the interview and two-week sleep diary. This laboratory protocol allows us to see whether the patient has an absence of sleep pathology (e.g., apnea, myoclonus, alpha–delta sleep) during his/her usual sleep period. If the patient initiates sleep considerably earlier than the sleep diary suggests, it is unlikely that the patient has a true delayed sleep phase. Rather, poor sleep hygiene and/or psychophysiological factors are probably playing a role in the disorder. Additional drug screens may be conducted just prior to each study to increase confidence of the polysomnographic results. A return visit is scheduled to discuss the results of the evaluation and sleep studies. Patients are asked to continue monitoring their sleep by keeping a sleep diary.

If a diagnosis of delayed sleep phase syndrome is confirmed by findings from the intake evaluation and polysomnographic data, a treatment approach is selected. Most of my experience has been with chronotherapy. This is a time-consuming, arduous procedure, but it is effective in resetting the circadian clock. All our delayed sleep phase syndrome patients are treated on an outpatient basis. In developing a treatment plan, I review the sleep diary data again and obtain information regarding average time of sleep onset and total sleep time. I also ask the patient what his/her desired sleep schedule is. With this information I proceed to develop a sleep schedule that is delayed three hours each day. Therefore, if a patient usually initiates sleep at 3:00 A.M. and sleeps a total of eight hours but desires a sleep schedule of 11:00 P.M. to 7:00 A.M., then he/she is to follow the schedule found in Table 1.

This protocol takes a total of eight days. During this time the patient often must take off from work or school. For treatment to be successful, it is extremely important that the patient and his/her family understand its rationale. I have found that some family members undermine the treatment even when it has been explained to them. Patients must be instructed to use a bedroom with little or no sunlight exposure. Construction paper taped to the windows acts as an inexpensive method of blocking out sunlight. The timing of meals is organized around the sleep periods. So despite the time of day, breakfast-type foods are always eaten during the first meal after awakening. Patients keep a record of their sleep behavior and call me daily to report on progress or problems. If they report an

Table 1. Sample Chronotherapy Schedule

Sleep period	In bed	Out of bed
1	3:00 A.M.	11:00 A.M.
2	6:00 A.M.	2:00 P.M.
3	9:00 A.M.	5:00 P.M.
4	12:00 P.M.	8:00 P.M.
5	3:00 P.M.	11:00 P.M.
6	6:00 P.M.	2:00 A.M.
7	9:00 P.M.	5:00 A.M.
8	11:00 P.M.	7:00 A.M.

inability to sleep at the prescribed hours, they are instructed to stay in the room and avoid environmental cues, if possible (e.g., sunlight). For several of my patients, having a video cassette player with several tapes to watch if they have difficulty sleeping has worked well.

Upon completion of chronotherapy, the patient returns for a follow-up visit. The importance of keeping the sleep schedule constant is stressed. Patients often ask, "How long do I have to keep this strict schedule? and "Can't I stay up late on weekends?" I usually make the analogy that just as some people can eat large amounts of food and not get fat while others eat large amounts of food and do get fat, so are there some people who can sleep at a variety of times and not be affected while others need regular bedtimes. "You are one of the latter people." I attempt to follow up each patient one month, three months, six months, and one year posttreatment. If problems arise and there has been a return to the delayed sleep period, chronotherapy can be repeated or another treatment may be added.

Interest in bright-light therapy has been focused on its effectiveness with patients who present with seasonal affective disorder. However, it can also be an effective treatment for delayed sleep phase syndrome. For a complete review of bright-light therapy see Terman (1989). Much of the reported success with bright light has been with 2500 lux of full-spectrum light. I use a light source that produces a light intensity of 10,000 lux. These light sources can be obtained commercially and are advertised in the pertinent journals and newsletters. We loan out the light box during the treatment phase. Given the difficulties associated with chronotherapy, bright-light therapy offers a promising alternative, but thus far I have treated only four patients with bright light. Utilizing the sleep diary and polysomnographic data, a schedule is developed for gradually waking earlier with 1.5 to 2 hours of exposure to bright light upon awakening. In my earlier example of the person who has an average sleep onset time of 3:00 A.M., the schedule shown in Table 2 would be presented and discussed.

This treatment can be as short as four nights; however, in several cases I have had to phase-advance only 15 minutes per night. In those cases

Table 2. Sample Bright-Light Schedule

Sleep period	In bed	Out of bed	Bright light
1	2:00 A.M.	10:00 A.M.	10 A.M.–12 A.M.
2	1:00 A.M.	9:00 A.M.	9 A.M.–11 A.M.
3	12:00 A.M.	8:00 P.M.	8 A.M.–10 A.M.
4	11:00 P.M.	7:00 A.M.	7 A.M.–9 A.M.

therapy took over two weeks. How long you must continue with bright light is based on the patient's report. I have found that a morning dose of 30 minutes at 10,000 lux can stabilize most patients. If they begin to drift (phase delay), an increased maintenance dosage can be recommended. Only recently have we begun to experiment with combined treatment of bright light and triazolam. We have tried this combined approach in only two patients who complained of difficulty initiating sleep after a phase advance was attempted with bright light. Only one of the patients appeared to benefit from administration of 0.25 mg triazolam two hours before the scheduled bedtime.

CASE STUDIES

A Successful Case

Mark, a 20-year-old man from a wealthy family, presented as an attractive, athletic-looking individual. He was a junior at a local state university, majoring in business. He lived at home with his mother and father. Mark was referred to the Sleep Disorders Center by a local neurologist. Prior to his consultation with the neurologist he had seen his family physician and a psychiatrist. Mark's primary problem was that he could not wake up in the morning. Over the years, Mark always had registered for afternoon classes; however, he needed to take two courses that were scheduled in the morning. He was failing these classes owing to absenteeism.

Mark reported that his parents always felt he was lazy because he could not wake up early in the morning. Left to his own schedule, he would sleep until 1:00 P.M. He labeled himself a "night owl" and stated that he enjoyed staying up and watching late-night television. This pattern reportedly began at about age 13. For years his mother and father would have to fight with him to wake up and go to school. His teachers reported that he often fell asleep in morning classes.

Mark attempted sleep at about 11:00 P.M. and got out of bed at 11:00 A.M. He slept until 1:00 P.M. on weekends. He usually did not initiate sleep until 3:00 A.M. His history was not suggestive of any other sleep pathology. However, Mark had a history of alcohol and drug abuse. Eight months ago he was hospitalized for four weeks for treatment of his chemical dependency. Besides alcohol, his other drug of choice was cocaine. Mark reported that since discharge from the hospital, he had no further periods of substance abuse or use. He smoked one pack of cigarettes per day. He drank six to eight caffeinated beverages per day. He exercised regularly, lifting weights primarily between 11:00 P.M. and 12:00 P.M., five nights per week. A complete physical examination conducted a month ago yielded no medical abnormalities. The drug screen conducted at the initial evaluation was negative.

On the MMPI, Mark had a valid profile. None of the clinical scales were elevated over a T-score of 70, suggesting that he was not suffering from significant psychopathology. However, a T-score of 68 was produced on the depression scale, indicating that he reported experiencing several symptoms of depression but not enough to suggest a mood disorder. Additionally, his T-score on the MacAndrew Alcoholism Scale was 70, which indicated a high risk for substance use or abuse. Mark denied being depressed but admitted to being very frustrated over his problem. Sleep diary data taken for three weeks prior to Mark's evaluation is presented in Table 3.

Polysomnography was conducted for two nights. On night 1, Mark was studied during his usual bedtime hours (11:45 P.M. to 11:00 A.M.). On night 2 he was studied during his sleep tendency period (3:00 A.M. to 11:00 A.M.) as determined by his sleep diary and self-report. Polysomnographic data is presented in Table 4.

From the evaluation and polysomnographic data, it was clear that Mark had a delayed sleep phase and fit the diagnostic criteria for delayed sleep phase syndrome. Treatment began with a discussion of sleep hygiene and how this might be improved. Specifically, I told Mark to decrease his caffeine intake, discontinue smoking at least one hour prior to his desired time of sleep onset, and reschedule his exercise earlier in the day. A course of chronotherapy delaying sleep three hours each sleep period was recommended. Mark's house has a guest room in the basement where there are no windows. It was decided that this would be the perfect place for him to undergo the chronotherapy schedule. Exposure to sunlight was to be avoided for two hours after awakening because sunlight is a powerful environmental stimulus which can inhibit or slow the ability to

Table 3. Sleep Diary Data for Mark (Three Weeks)

Mean time of sleep attempt	11:30 P.M.
Mean time of sleep onset	3:15 A.M.
Mean time of final awakening	11:12 A.M.
Mean time in bed	11.74 hours
Mean sleep latency	3.75 hours
Mean total sleep time	7.34 hours
Mean wake after sleep onset	40 minutes
Mean sleep efficiency	62.5 percent

Table 4. Polysomnographic Data on Mark

A.M.	Night 1 11:45 P.M.–11:00 A.M.	Night 2 3:00 A.M.–11:00 P.M.
Sleep efficiency	64 percent	85 percent
Sleep-onset latency	4.05 hours	1.2 hours
Total sleep time	7.2 hours	6.8 hours
REM latency	97 minutes	72 minutes

Summary: The patient did not demonstrate any breathing, cardiac, or electrocardiogrraphic abnormalities.

delay further. An attempt was made to engage his parents in the process, but Mark did not want them involved. He wanted to demonstrate his independence by solving the problem without their aid.

Mark was successful with the chronotherapy. He took 10 days off from school but used his time during treatment to study for upcoming exams. To aid in his entrainment, I recommended exposure to sunlight upon awakening for 30 minutes to an hour. A longer exposure time was more desirable (e.g., two hours); however, Mark's schedule did not allow for this. At his three-month follow-up, Mark was doing well. He reported having moderate difficulty concentrating in the morning; however, he had passed all his courses. At the six-month follow-up, Mark reported that he had returned to his delayed sleep schedule. Over the summer he stayed up late for four nights in a row and could not return to the advanced schedule. He repeated the chronotherapy treatment successfully. At one-year follow-up, his schedule was beginning to drift and I recommended he purchase a set of bright lights for morning exposure. He was to expose himself to the bright lights one hour immediately upon awakening. When I contacted Mark recently, he was about to graduate from college. He had been able to stabilize his sleep period successfully with no return to the delayed sleep schedule.

An Unsuccessful Case

Leslie, a 17-year-old high-school senior, lived with her mother. Her mother was recently divorced and Leslie did not have any contact with her father. She had no brothers or sisters. Leslie's mother read an article about the Sleep Disorders Center in the paper and asked her family physician to make a referral. Leslie presented to the Sleep Disorders Center as a slender woman with a complaint of insomnia and daytime sleepiness. She had missed 40 days of school this year and was in danger of failing her senior year. In general, Leslie was a bright student making mainly A's and B's. At the time of the evaluation Leslie appeared depressed. She cried periodically and stated that she felt like a failure. A recent move to Tennessee had reportedly been difficult for her. She had many friends in North Carolina but was having trouble making friends in the new school.

The sleep problem reportedly began 1.5 years ago. She began staying up late to work on school assignments. Her mother underwent a daily struggle to wake her up to make it to the school bus on time. School performance remained good. A pattern of insomnia developed. She attempted sleep at 10:30 P.M. but could not get to sleep until 2:30 A.M. Sleep onset did not usually occur until 3:30 A.M. If not for her mother's insistence, she slept until 12:30 P.M. and to 2:30 P.M. on weekends. Leslie's sleep diary data is presented in Table 5.

Polysomnography was conducted for two nights using our standard protocol. This data is presented in Table 6. A pattern of delayed sleep phase syndrome was confirmed.

On the MMPI, Leslie had a valid profile. Elevations of scales 2 (depression) and 3 (hysteria) over T-scores of 70 suggested significant psychological distress. I decided to refer Leslie for a psychiatric evaluation, and a course of antidepressant medication with weekly psychotherapy was tried. I suggested to Leslie that her depression needed to improve before we began treatment for her delayed sleep phase.

Leslie returned in ten weeks and was anxious to begin chronotherapy treatment, as there had been no improvement in her ability to initiate sleep at the desired bedtime. Her depression had improved significantly; however, she remained unable to wake in the morning. The standard chronotherapy treatment was employed. On sleep periods 1 to 3, she had no difficulty; however, she called on day 4 to report she could not go on with treatment because is interfered with her work schedule and she feared losing her job. Despite the fact that this problem had been anticipated and discussed, she decided to quit the chronotherapy.

Table 5. Sleep Diary Data for Leslie (Two Weeks)

Mean time of sleep attempt	10:45 P.M.
Mean time of sleep onset	3:25 A.M.
Mean time of final awakening	12:40 P.M.
Mean time in bed	13.92 hours
Mean sleep latency	4.66 hours
Mean total sleep time	8.65 hours
Mean wake after sleep onset	37 minutes
Mean sleep efficiency	60 percent

Table 6. Polysomnographic Data on Leslie

	Night 1 (11:00 P.M.–11:30 A.M.)	Night 2 (3:15 A.M.–11:30 A.M.)
Sleep efficiency	55 percent	92 percent
Sleep-onset latency	4.66 hours	0.66 hour
Total sleep time	6.84 hours	7.6 hours
REM latency	64 minutes	52 minutes

Summary: The patient did not demonstrate any breathing, cardiac, or electrocardiographic abnormalities.

Leslie returned two months later and asked for help in beginning chronotherapy again. A new schedule was developed and she seemed determined to follow through. Four days later I received a call from Leslie's mother reporting that Leslie could not comply with the treatment regime and they decided not to return for additional follow-up. Some patients may report an inability to tolerate the chronotherapy schedule. In Leslie's case I believe that depression continued to be a problem interfering with her ability to tolerate and adapt to the continually changing sleep–wake schedule. If Leslie returns, I may try a course of bright-light treatment.

Russell Rosenberg received his Ph.D. in Clinical Psychology from the Ohio State University in 1986. He served as director of St. Mary's Sleep Disorders Center in Knoxville, Tennessee for four years. He also held an appointment as Assistant Professor of Psychology at the University of Tennessee. Currently Dr. Rosenberg is director of Northside Hospital's Sleep Disorders Center in Atlanta, Georgia, and is a fellow of the American Sleep Disorders Association.

RECOMMENDED READINGS

Czeisler, C. A., Richardson, G. S., Coleman, R. M., Zimmerman, J. C., Moore-Ede, M. C., Dement, W. C., & Weitzman, E. D. (1981). Chronotherapy: Resetting the circadian clocks of patients with delayed sleep phase insomnia. *Sleep, 4,* 1–21.
The authors describe their treatment of five delayed sleep phase syndrome patients with chronotherapy. A rationale for using chronotherapy as a treatment for delayed sleep phase insomniacs is discussed.

Morris, M., Lack, L., & Dawson, D. (1990). Sleep onset insomniacs have delayed temperature rhythms. *Sleep, 13,* 1–14.
This article presents a brief review of circadian rhythms as they pertain to sleep-onset insomnia. The authors suggest that many sleep-onset insomniacs may have less extreme cases of delayed sleep phase syndrome. Implications for treatment and possible causes for phase delay are discussed.

REFERENCES

Coleman, R. M., Roffwarg, H. P., Kennedy, S. V., Guilleminault, C., Cinque, J., Cohn, M. A., Karacan, I., Kupfer, D. J., Lemmi, H., Miles, L. E., Orr, E. C., Phillips, E. R., Roth, T., Sassin, J. F., Schmidt, H., & Dement, W. C. (1982). Sleep–wake disorders based on a polysomnographic diagnosis: A national cooperative study. *Journal of the American Medical Association, 247,* 997–1003.

Czeisler, C. A., Richardson, G. S., Coleman, R. M., Zimmerman, J. C., Moore-Ede, M. C., Dement, W. C., & Weitzman, E. D. (1981). Chronotherapy: Resetting the circadian clocks of patients with delayed sleep phase insomnia. *Sleep, 4,* 1–21.

Lewy, A. J., Singer, C. M., & Sack, R. L., (1985). Treatment of appropriately phase typed sleep disorders using properly timed light. *Sleep Research, 14,* 304.

Mendelson, W. (1987). *Human sleep: Research and clinical care.* New York: Plenum Press.

Pelayo, R. P., Thorpy, M. J., & Glovinsky, P. (1988). Prevalence of delayed sleep phase syndrome among adolescents. *Sleep Research, 17,* 391.

Piercy, J., & Lack, L. (1988). Daily exercise can shift the endogenous circadian phase. *Sleep Research, 17,* 393.

Terman, M. (1989). Light therapy. In M. H. Kryger, T. Roth, & W. C. Dement (Eds.), *Principles and practice of sleep medicine.* Philadelphia: W. B. Saunders, pp. 717–722.

Uruha, S., Mikami, V. S. Teshima, Y., Sugita, Y., Honda, H., Inatani, K., Taehibana, N., Egawa, I., Tsutsumi, T., & Iijima, S. (1987). Effect of triazolam for delayed sleep phase syndrome. *Sleep Research, 16,* 650.

Vanderpool, J. R. J., Kelly, K. G., Schultz, P. M., Allen, R., Souetre, E., & Rosenthal, N. E. (1988). Delayed sleep phase syndrome revisited: Preliminary effects of light and triazolam. *Sleep Research, 17,* 381.

Vanderpool, J. R. J., Rosenthal, N. E., Levendosky, A. A., Johnson, S. H., Allen, R., Kelly, K. A., Soutre, E., Schultz, P. M., & Stafz, K. (1989). Phase shifting effects of bright morning light as treatment for delayed sleep phase syndrome. *Sleep Research, 18,* 422.

Weitzman, E. D., Czeisler, C. A., Coleman, R. M., Spielman, A. J., Zimmerman, J. C., & Dement, W. C., (1981). Delayed sleep phase syndrome: A chronological disorder with sleep onset insomnia. *Archives of General Psychiatry, 38,* 737–746.

Wever, R. A. (1979). *The circadian system of man.* New York: Springer-Verlag.

CHAPTER THIRTEEN

Early Morning Awakening Insomnia
Bright-Light Treatment

RICHARD P. ALLEN

INTRODUCTION

This chapter's title may seem a bit odd. It focuses on a little-used treatment concept for insomnia—exposure to bright light and its application for a type of insomnia commonly associated with depression and/or old age—namely early morning awakening (EMA). The EMA symptom is usually assumed to indicate depression and therefore sometimes receives scant consideration in sleep disorders medicine. Similarly, bright-light treatment has become associated with winter depression (seasonal affective disorder) (Rosenthal et al., 1984) and sometimes with transitory management of abrupt changes in circadian rhythm (Daan & Lewy, 1984) and is not usually considered in the management of chronic insomnia. Indeed, the most recent major text on sleep disorders medicine (Kryger, Roth, & Dement, 1989) does not even include a reference to this type of treatment for persistent insomnia. Moreover, when light treatment is considered for chronic insomnia, it is usually reserved for sleep-onset insomnia associated with early morning sleepiness (Pittendrigh, 1981), essentially the reverse symptom of that considered here. The following discussion and case are presented because they illustrate some of the potential advantages and indications for adding bright-light treatment to the treatment of EMA.

Richard P. Allen • Sleep Disorders Center, Johns Hopkins University School of Medicine, Baltimore, Maryland 21224.

The clinical rationale for the treatment described here stems from the chronobiology both of the target symptom and of bright-light treatment.

EMA SYMPTOM

The classical differential diagnosis for insomnia emphasizes the time during the sleep period disturbed by waking. Sleep-onset insomnia indicates excessive wake time at sleep onset or during the first part of sleep; sleep maintenance insomnia indicates excessive wake time after sleep is established. The sleep maintenance insomnias are subdivided by awakenings occurring throughout sleep versus awakenings occurring mostly in the last half of sleep during the early morning. The latter syndrome is called early morning awakening in this chapter. EMA is sometimes subdivided into sleep with premature awakening without return to sleep versus sleep with frequent early awakenings with a return to sleep; both these symptoms are considered appropriate for the treatment presented here.

EMA SYMPTOMS AND DIFFERENTIAL DIAGNOSIS

EMA relates to three primary diagnostic conditions. Foremost among these is primary affective disorder (depression). Depression in affective disorder classically produces EMA, not uncommonly with sleepiness in the evening and little or no other disturbance of sleep. Depression when present with other symptoms should always be treated as the primary disorder; however, milder depressive reactions may occur in which the sleep disorder may be more severe and disabling than other symptoms. The mechanisms producing the sleep disturbance symptoms in a major depressive disorder appear to be also involved in other aspects of psychologically disturbed behavior without significant depression. It is tempting to assume there is some underlying depression in most of the more severe EMA conditions; this is often not clinically validated. Moreover, jumping to antidepressant medications presents significant risks and avoids the possibility that more effective treatments might be used with less risk. Therefore, the pharmacological management of depression should be reserved for cases where diagnosis meets the classical criteria for a major depression disorder and, in particular, where the EMA is not the primary disturbing symptom. Similarly, the psychological treatments for depression, such as cognitive therapies, may ignore treatment of the sleep disorder and may fail to reduce the rather marked suffering experienced from chronic insomnia. For dysthymia or personality disorder, with a major disturbing symptom of EMA, a more direct focus on symptom treatment, such as described below, may be appropriate in addition to other psychological treatments.

The second condition causing EMA is anxiety awakenings, usually related to awakening from early morning dreams, which tend to be more intense and involve more emotional content than dreams during the first part of sleep. These awakenings are often accompanied by dream content, although sometimes only the timing of the awakenings and the report of anxiety on awakening suggest the relationship to anxious thoughts during sleep. For severely disturbing dreams, the dream content itself may need to be addressed in therapy, perhaps using dream completion therapy techniques or therapy directed at resolving the conflicts related to the anxiety. When these awakenings are accompanied by significant daytime anxiety symptoms, treatment of the overall anxiety disorder with medications and psychotherapy should be considered as the primary treatment focus. In the absence of significant wake-time anxiety symptoms the anxiety awakenings may be considered as indicating a time of night vulnerable to awakening. The awakenings could result from either increased stimulus to arouse or decreased threshold for arousal occurring during these times. EMA from increased stimuli to arouse occurring in the later part of the sleep cycle might lead to sleepiness early in the evening. This could eventually produce a sleep cycle disturbance reducing arousal thresholds in the morning and increasing susceptibility to arousing stimuli, thereby exacerbating the condition. Bright-light treatment could reduce arousal thresholds during this vulnerable time. This could reduce the awakening response to the arousal stimuli and improve sleep. The anxiety caused by fear of the awakening would then be reduced by a bright-light treatment.

Sleep–wake cycle disturbance is the EMA-related condition for which the light treatment should be considered the treatment of choice. Sleepiness is controlled by two separate neurological mechanisms—one related to maintaining a homeostasis for balancing the amount of time spent asleep with that spent awake, and the other related to maintaining a daily cycle of sleep and waking corresponding to the light–dark cycle. The homeostasis specifies the desired amount of sleep in any 24-hour cycle and is shown profoundly by the effects of sleep deprivation increasing depth and amount of subsequent sleep. The circadian cycle of sleepiness is demonstrated most profoundly by the problems people experience with wakefulness despite adequate sleep following transmeridian airplane travel ("jet lag") or when working nightshifts.

The circadian rhythm of activity in primates appears to be controlled by the suprachiasmatic nuclei, which are necessary and sufficient for maintaining this basic circadian rhythm independent of external cues (Fuller, Lydic, Sulzman, Albers, Tepper, & Moore-Ede, 1981; Stephan & Zucker, 1972). The primary neurological mechanisms controlling the basic circadian activity rhythm can operate independently of external cues. Ideally, onset of the sleep phase of this biological circadian cycle corresponds to desired bedtimes (usually late evening; e.g., 10:30 P.M.), with onset of the wake phase corresponding to desired time for awakening (usually in the morning; e.g., 6:30 A.M.). The timing of this cycle will vary with individual social demands but needs to be relatively stable. Adjustments to changes generally require about one to two days for each two to four hours of change in schedule.

Problems develop when the biological circadian cycle is out of phase with social demands. Thus, the sleep phase could be delayed relative to social demands; i.e., the person becomes sleepy only much after the desired bedtime (sleep-onset problems) and becomes alert only much after the desired awakening time (morning sleepiness) (Weitzman, Czeisler, Coleman, Spielman, Zimmerman, & Dement, 1981). Alternatively, the sleep phase could be advanced with an early onset of sleepiness in the evening (evening sleepiness) and an early onset of wakefulness in the morning (EMA). EMA could, therefore, result from a sleep phase advance syndrome—characterized by evening sleepiness and EMA persisting for several months despite attempts at keeping a regular schedule with little evening sleep. This condition could lead to sufficient sleep loss to produce a sense of sleepiness throughout most of the day, but the sleepiness would be most severe in the evening and least during the morning.

BRIGHT LIGHTS AND THE SLEEP-WAKE CYCLE

The biological circadian rhythm corresponds to the light-dark cycle, with sleepiness during the dark phase for humans. In the absence of any external cues, this cycle persists with a cycle length of about 25 to 28 hours for humans. That is, without external cues the sleep-wake cycle for humans is generally longer than 24 hours. External cues are used to continually reset this cycle to our 24-hour light-dark cycle. Classical work had shown that for almost all species, the primary external stimuli for setting this cycle is exposure to light (Rusak & Zucker, 1975). For humans, however, early work had erroneously shown no effect of light on the circadian rhythm, and it had, therefore been assumed that the primary stimuli for humans were social cues. Later work by Czeisler, Weitzman, and others, however, showed that humans, indeed, respond to light—but unlike other animals, they require a very bright light, exceeding 2500 lux, to produce a significant change in the circadian rhythm (Czeisler *et al.*, 1986; Czeisler, Richardson, Zimmerman, Moore-Ede, & Weitzman, 1981). Thus humans, like other animals, have a mechanism that responds to external light for resetting the circadian rhythm, but the amount of light required is greater than had been expected. Similarly, it has been shown that humans' response to light, like that of other mammals, depends on when in the sleep–wake cycle the light is presented. Basically, bright light presented at the time of the awakening in the biological sleep–wake cycle (an artificially early dawn) produces an advance in the biological sleep phase. Essentially, this advance compensates for the unexpectedly early dawn by moving the sleep time earlier. Conversely, bright light presented at the time of sleepiness in the biological sleep—wake cycle (an artificially late dusk) produces a delay in the biological sleep phase. This delay compensates for the unexpectedly late end to the daytime by moving the sleep phase later.

As Rosenberg discusses in Chapter Twelve, the delayed sleep cycle syndrome can be corrected by morning bright-light treatment. This produces a change in the sleep phase to earlier times (sleep phase advance). The duration of exposure to the light and the intensity of the light both serve to change the effect on the sleep phase. Longer exposure and brighter intensity both increase the effect. Light exposure past the awakening phase of the cycle has diminishing effects and, of course, when continued into the period shortly before the onset of the sleep phase, has a counterproductive effect serving to again delay the sleep phase and restoring the pathology. To avoid this counterproductive effect of afternoon and evening light, patients with sleep phase delay are asked to wear very dark, wraparound sunglasses (miner's goggles or mountaineer's glasses) after 4:00 P.M. whenever they are in sunlight.

The advanced sleep phase syndrome with EMA is expected to respond to the reverse treatment given for the sleep phase delay. That is, bright evening light and dark goggles in the morning should produce a delay in the sleep phase so that sleep lasts longer into the morning. The expected effect is actually even a bit more general. The degree of sleepiness changes with the core body temperature; sleepiness is maximal at the low point of the temperature cycle and decreases in relation to increasing temperature. The temperature minimum is advanced by evening light. With that advance there is a decrease in arousal threshold during the morning. In this way, at least in theory, evening light can be used to reduce vulnerability to EMA even in conditions when sleep cycle advance is not clearly evident, provided problems do not develop with either sleep onset or morning sleepiness after awakening.

Despite these strong theoretical bases for use of bright light to treat EMA, it has not been experimentally verified. The following case is a successful example of its application and demonstrates, in general, how light treatment may be used for some insomnia conditions. Adequate experimental verification of the validity of this approach is, unfortunately, not currently available.

CASE HISTORY

Presenting Complaint

Mr. M, a 43-year-old, white male professional, was referred by his family doctor to the Hopkins Sleep Disorder Center with a five-year history of premature EMA, usually from 2:00 to 4:00 A.M., accompanied by some anxious ruminating thoughts. Mr. M was also usually very sleepy during the evening.

History of Present Illness

Mr. M had few sleep problems until about six years ago when he developed, over a period of a few months, a profound insomnia with EMA and on some occasions only a brief two to four hours of sleep followed by a premature awakening without return to sleep. He complained of work-related stress with feelings of anxiety, doubts about his ability to adequately perform his job, particularly after a poor night's sleep, and persistent intrusive, ruminating thoughts about his work disrupting his sleep at night. He reported loss of concentration, crying spells, suicidal thoughts, hopelessness, or even very evident sad periods.

About 6 to 12 months after the problem started, Mr. M was hospitalized for one week with a diagnosis of major depressive disorder. He was discharged to outpatient therapy with his depression and anxiety lessened but his insomnia persisting. His medication treatments included various antidepressants; these were discontinued owing to iimited benefit and unpleasant side effects developing at the usual therapeutic doses. Xanax (0.25 to 0.5 mg) was also prescribed for EMA to facilitate return to sleep; this had been continued fairly regularly for two to five days a week throughout much of the past four years. During this time he was also engaged in various outpatient therapies, carrying the diagnoses of depression and passive/dependent personality.

Mr. M's psychotherapy included cognitive and behavioral therapies. He experienced marked improvement in his depression without any significant improvement in the insomnia. He reported that the only medication that helped his insomnia in the doses he could tolerate was the Xanax and that without Xanax he would frequently get less than four hours sleep a night. He complained of daytime sleepiness much worse in the evening; this had become so bad that at times he found himself falling asleep while driving a car. Throughout this time he was judged by his supervisors as having an excellent to outstanding work performance; there was no indication that his ability to work was disrupted aside from problems associated with sleepiness mostly during the latter part of the day.

Sleep Patterns at the Time of Evaluation

Mr. M typically went to bed at approximately 11:00 P.M. and fell asleep rapidly, but he awakened around 2:00 to 4:00 A.M. After awakening he would start thinking about work problems and sometimes would become very involved in solving or worrying about these problems. As noted, he would take Xanax about two or three times a week to return to sleep after an awakening. He would always lie in bed until about 6:30 to 7:00 A.M. and then he would get up to start the day.

Medical History

Medical history was significant for hiatal hernia with occasional heartburn, which improved with the use of bethanecol (Urecholine). A trial on metoclopramide (Reglan) had dramatically exacerbated the daytime sleepiness and was discontinued. Mr. M also had bronchial asthma, exercise-induced cough, and dyspnea with a good response to provental inhaler. Trials off bethanecol led to significant recurrence of reflux and it was therefore continued despite the asthma problems. At the time of this evaluation he was taking only the bethanecol, 10 mg three times daily, and Xanax, 0.5 mg three to four times per week, on EMA.

At this time Mr. M was 71 inches tall, weighed 178 pounds, and was normal on physical, psychiatric, and neurological examination. He did not smoke cigarettes, denied drug abuse, and drank little alcohol.

Personal History

Mr. M had a stable marriage of 21 years; he had four children and a working wife. He had a successful professional career and reported no significant family problems or real work-related problems aside from his self-imposed pressure for success.

Family History

Mr. M's mother was reported to have been treated for depression. His father had loud snoring and some daytime sleepiness.

Laboratory Sleep Tests

A polysomnogram and a multiple sleep latency test were obtained with the patient off Xanax for over ten days. The test showed rapid sleep onset and normal REM–NREM cycles, with a total sleep time of 366 minutes and sleep efficiency of 98 percent. Mr. M had only minimal wake after sleep onset (5.5 minutes), which occurred in the early morning. He showed no significant abnormal movements in sleep. He had mild hypopneas during sleep occurring at a rate of about 19 per hour for about 19 percent of the sleep time, with little oxygen desaturation (O_2SAT: baseline 97 percent, minimum 92 percent). Few (36 percent) of these events were associated with arousals. We considered the sleep-related hypopneas to have little clinical significance. The multiple sleep latency test the next day showed normal sleep latencies greater than 13 minutes for tests at 9:00 A.M., 11:00 A.M., and 1:00 P.M.; the test at 3:00 P.M. had a sleep latency of five minutes. Mr. M reported he slept much better in the lab than at home.

Treatment and Added Diagnostic Studies

After the essentially normal sleep laboratory evaluation, we referred the patient for further psychiatric evaluation. Sleep hygiene was also discussed with an emphasis on continuing off Xanax and other sleep-related medications, avoiding naps, and not using alcohol in the evening because of possible exacerbation of the sleep-related hypopnea. At the patient's request, a further review of his symptoms led to a one-week activity monitoring of the home sleep pattern using a wrist activity monitor. This showed bedtimes of 11:00 P.M. to 7:00 A.M. disturbed by EMA, with total sleep times of about 4.5 to 6 hours, similar to that reported by the patient for his usual sleep at home and worse than that in the sleep laboratory. Treatment as detailed below was, therefore, started with an initial trial on a sleep restriction protocol. Only after that had essentially failed was bright-light therapy attempted.

Sleep Restriction Treatment. Mr. M's baseline week of self-reported sleep showed usual sleep times of 11:00 P.M. to 7:00 A.M. with an average of 4.5 hours sleep (54 percent sleep efficiency). This was considered by him to be a fairly usual week. He was then put on the usual sleep restriction regime (see Chapter Four) with bedtimes starting at 1:30 to 7:00 A.M. He reported a worsening of symptoms over the next four days, with decreased sleep time and little change in his ability to stay asleep in the early morning. After a few days he broke the routine with a return to 11:30 P.M. bedtime, which he then agreed to further delay until 12:00 A.M. for a schedule of 12:00 to 7:00 A.M. sleep. He was unwilling to try to further delay his sleep times.

Mr. M was away on vacation with little improvement in sleep, but on return he accepted an 11:30 P.M. to 6:30 A.M. sleep time goal. On this he achieved about a 75 percent sleep efficiency, with an average of about 5.25 hours of sleep. He considered this a modest improvement and reluctantly agreed to a further restriction in bedtimes to 12:00 to 6:00 A.M. He developed a slightly improved sleep efficiency with no change in total sleep time. When bedtime was advanced to 11:45 P.M., he showed essentially no change in total sleep time and he was unable to achieve a better sleep efficiency. He felt only mild improvement in sleep with this treatment and was not satisfied with the degree of improvement.

Bright-Light Treatment. Treatment was continued with the addition of artificial bright lights (2500 lux) to be used from 8:00 to 10:00 P.M. and wearing dark, wraparound sunglasses whenever outside from awakening to noon. The lights were used in such a fashion that they shone directly on the eyes from a lightbox placed on a desk within two feet of the patient's head. (Looking directly at the lights is not required, but the eyes must not be shaded from the lights.) For this treatment the patient bought a commercially available set of lights. He was also continued on the mildly restricted sleep schedule with bedtimes from 12:00 to 6:30 A.M.

Within the first two weeks on this treatment, sleep time improved to an average of six hours per night, with a reported decrease in EMA. This was the first time that the patient felt that EMA were decreasing and he reported that the lights were helping him. A short trial off the lights showed a return to poorer sleep, with sleep times of 4.5 to 5.0 hours. His time in bed was then extended to 11:30 P.M. to 7:00 A.M. and continued on that schedule for four weeks. For the last week he reported an average sleep time of 6.5 hours, with a subjective report of good to very good sleep.

A follow-up evaluation five months latter indicated continued use of the lights with good to very good sleep and 6.5 to 7 hours of sleep on most nights. Bed times were 11:00 P.M. to 7:00 A.M. This was reported to be the first time the patient felt reasonably free of EMA in the past five years. Sleepiness in the evening also decreased.

DISCUSSION

The case described here demonstrates merely that bright-light treatment for sleep phase advance is practical and might work. In this particular case the bright-light treatment was essentially tried as a treatment of almost last resort. Despite the bitter complaints of the patient regarding his sleep, he showed fairly normal sleep in the sleep laboratory. This problem of discrepancy between sleep complaint and sleep lab findings is not uncommon; the patient's clinical report, including the daytime sleepiness, was convincing and we felt a further objective evaluation would help. We therefore obtained a week-long wrist activity monitor, which demonstrated the poor sleep reported by the patient. This provided objective documentation that in his home environment his normal sleep patterns were very disturbed, contrary to the conclusion we had reached from the laboratory study. We were then left with a dilemma regarding treatment. After five years of psychotherapy and multiple psychiatric consultation, yet another referral for psychiatric evaluation hardly seemed promising. We had successfully treated other patients with major insomnia complaints using the sleep restriction approach and it seemed a reasonable approach for this case. The sleep restriction trial was frustrating both because of the limited cooperation from the patient and because of the stubborn persistence of the EMA in the face of significant decrease in prior sleep; at this point we started to seriously consider this problem as, in part, a sleep phase advance. We already had reason to suspect that forced schedule changes do not themselves alter the sleep–wake cycle, particularly for those patients having a sleep phase disturbance.

It was, however, only the patient's subjective response to the bright lights that caused us to review the history and then see everywhere the rather marked evidence for a sleep phase advance: EMA, early evening sleepiness, resistance of EMA to sleep schedule changes, no improvement in sleep on holidays, no depressed mood, no disruption of work except for that related to sleepiness, and poor response to medications. All of these now suggest a sleep phase advance syndrome—always clearer with hindsight.

This patient's report of a continuing need to use the lights is similar to the results from the sleep phase delay study (Rosenthal *et al.*, 1990). These patients seem to be unable to maintain their adjustment to socially defined sleep–wake schedules without added signals for resetting the biological circadian rhythm. This result suggests there is some abnormality disrupting the normal relationship between the patients' biological circadian rhythm and external cues or possibly a biological circadian cycle shorter than normal. It remains to be seen if this abnormality corrects with longer-term use of the bright-light treatment or if some form of fading from the lights might be successful in correcting this problem. At this point, however, it can be expected that for these cases the use of the lights may be required for at least several weeks or months.

The treatment response to bright lights was slower in this case than I might have expected, but I am not convinced that the patient sat under the light for a full two hours, and the response would undoubtedly have been better if a much brighter light, up to 10,000 lux, had been used. These brighter lights are now available and I recommend their use; the 2500 lux appears to be marginal for producing the desired change. Moreover, the duration of exposure can be compromised more with the brighter lights.

The significance of the dark wraparound sunglasses is theoretical, but for a sleep phase advance problem, avoiding the morning sunlight may be very important. We have not evaluated this is any systematic fashion, but generally have been pleased with the acceptance from our patients of the use of these glasses. They can be readily obtained from major sporting-goods stores.

It's the large box of lights which causes the most problems. These lights need to be purchased or rented from one of several companies now handling such devices. In our experience, some of the major medical equipment rental companies will provide these for a short-term trial rental (current cost of about $100 for two weeks), but it appears that the units would need to be purchased by the patient for longer-term use (current cost $300 to $600). The use of the lights is somewhat awkward for the patient. Some patients complain of glare from the lights, particularly for the 10,000-lux lights, which are designed for the patient to be closer to the light than for the 2500-lux lights. In our experience, the problem of glare or discomfort from the lights has been minimal. A more significant problem has been arranging the time for the patient to sit under the lights. In this regard, treatment of the advanced sleep phase is somewhat more easily accepted than the delayed sleep phase as the evening times when the lights are to be used are usually private times at home. In contrast, the morning times (when lights are used for the delayed sleep cycle condition) are generally more rushed, with little personal time. Adding a two-hour block of personal time to the morning can be socially difficult, while adding this time in the evening is generally more acceptable. We explain to the patient that the time chosen to be under the lights is already generally compromised by sleepiness and therefore this is not a loss of quality time. Some activity such as reading or crafts activity is recommended while under the lights to help maintain wakefulness. For a professional, as in this case, the time with the lights is often used for reading or writing. For this it needs to be emphasized that the lights must shine on the eyes; illumination of materials being read is not a significant aspect of the treatment.

This case raises the interesting issue of the relationship between depression and sleep phase advance. Many depressed patients report sleep phase advance symptoms but usually as only one of the symptoms. This particular case presented with clear, dramatic symptoms of sleep cycle advance with no sleep-onset problems, profound EMA, and significant evening sleepiness. The symptoms for a major depression other than EMA were less evident and, indeed, this diagnosis was made only during the short hospitalization. In fact, wake-time depression symptoms for this patient were rather few aside from those related to sleepiness and anxiety about falling asleep. Nonetheless, the ruminating, anxious thoughts on awakening were seen as strongly suggesting an underlying anxiety or depressive disorder causing the EMA; this was further supported by the positive family history for depression. With hindsight it is tempting to suggest that correction of the sleep phase advance would have corrected the EMA, leaving the patient free of the anxious morning thoughts. This, however, seems unlikely. It is more likely that there were two problems in this case, each needing separate consideration: excessive anxiety regarding work performance and an advanced sleep phase. Sleep disorders medicine offers light treatment for the advanced sleep phase syndrome. When the sleep disturbance is as pronounced a symptom as in this case, this treatment may be considered, if for no other reason than it will serve to reduce the ease with which the patient's sleep can be disturbed during the morning sleep.

While the bright-light treatment approach seems promising, it remains to be experimentally validated. The results in a case like this may represent placebo or response demand effects. Prior failure to respond to other treatments may have improved the possibility of responding to this different, more direct approach to the sleep problem, although the failure to respond to sleep restriction argues against a response demand interpretation. Nonetheless, until we have better experimental validation of this treatment for the sleep phase advance, it should be undertaken cautiously, recognizing the experimental nature of the treatment. Without better experimental data, the light treatment cannot be considered an adequate complete treatment for any condition with psychological disturbance, but it can be cautiously offered as part of a treatment plan in conjunction with other treatments.

SUMMARY OF TREATMENT APPROACH

Diagnostic procedures
  History: medical, psychological, family, sleep
  Physical examination
  Mental status examination
  Polysomnogram
  Multiple sleep latency test
  Activity monitor (wrist movements over seven days)
Advanced sleep phase syndrome:
  Awakenings, disturbing sleep in second half of the sleep
  First half of the sleep relatively undisturbed
  No significant disturbance of sleep onset
  Early evening sleepiness excessive and greater than any sleepiness in the morning
  Persistence for several months (more than six)

Persistence despite attempts to change schedule
Disruptive of desired life activities
Not secondary to concurrent major depression
Bright-light treatment for sleep phase advance
Regular sleep–wake schedule (11:00 P.M. to 7:00 A.M.) with no naps
Bright lights (>2500 lux) for two hours in late evening (8:00 to 11:00 P.M.)
Dark, wraparound sunglasses (mountaineer's) worn from morning awakening until noon
Response occurs within two weeks
May need to be continued to avoid relapse

Richard P. Allen is a clinical psychologist in the Department of Neurology at the Johns Hopkins University School of Medicine. He received his B.S. degree in Mathematics from M.I.T. and his Ph.D. in Psychology from the University of Cambridge, England. He started the Sleep Disorders Center at Johns Hopkins and is codirector of the center. He has worked with a wide variety of insomnia problems, including restless legs, periodic limb movements in sleep, and circadian rhythm disorders. His recent work includes collaboration with the National Institute of Mental Health on a controlled research evaluation of bright-light treatment for the delayed sleep phase syndrome.

RECOMMENDED READINGS

Dinges, D. F. (1989). The influence of the human circadian timekeeping system on sleep. In M. H. Kryger, T. Roth, & W. C. Dement (Eds.), *Principles and practice of sleep medicine*. Philadelphia: W. B. Saunders, Chapter 12, pp. 153–162.
A good review of the relationship between chronobiology and human sleep.
Moore-Ede, M.C., Sulzman, F. M., & Fuller, C. A. (1982). *The clocks that time us*. Cambridge, MA: Harvard University Press.
A good technical review of chronobiology.
Terman, M. (1989). Light therapy. In M. H. Kryger, T. Roth & W. C. Dement (Eds.), *Principles and practice of sleep medicine*. Philadelphia: W. B. Saunders, Chapter 78, pp. 717–722.
Tells how to use bright lights for seasonal adaptation disorder.

REFERENCES

Czeisler, C. A., Allan, J. S., Storogatz, S. H., Ronda, J. M., Sánchez, R., Rios, C. D., Freitag, W. O., Richardson, G. S., & Kronauer, R. E. (1986). Bright light resets the human circadian pacemaker independent of the timing of the sleep-wake cycle. *Science, 233*, 667–671.

Czeisler, C. A., Richardson, G. S., Zimmerman, J. C., Moore-Ede, M. C., & Weitzman, E. D. (1981). Entrainment of human circadian rhythms by light–dark cycles: A reassessment. *Photochemical Photobiology, 34*, 239–247.

Daan, S., & Lewy, A. J. (1984). Scheduled exposure to daylight: A potential strategy to reduce "jet lag" following transmeridian flight. *Psychopharmacological Bulletin, 20*, 566–568.

Fuller, C. A., Lydic, R., Sulzman, F. M., Albers, H. E., Tepper, B., & Moore-Ede, M. C. (1981). Circadian rhythm of body temperature persists after suprachiasmatic lesions in the squirrel monkey. *American Journal of Physiology, 241*, R385–R391.

Kryger, M. H., Roth, T., & Dement, W. C. (1989). *Principals and practice of sleep medicine.* Philadelphia: W. B. Saunders, p. 739.

Pittendrigh, C. S. (1981). Circadian systems: Entrainment. In J. Aschoff (Ed.), *Handbook of behavioral biology: Biological rhythms*. New York: Plenum Press, pp. 95–124.

Rosenthal, N. E., Joseph-Vanderpool, J. R., Levendosky, A. A., Johnston, S. H., Allen, R. P., Kelly, K. A., Souetre, E., Schulz, P. M., & Starz, K. E. (1990). Phase-shifting effects of bright morning light treatment for delayed sleep phase syndrome. *Sleep, 13*, 354–361.

Rosenthal, N. E., Sack, D. A., Gillin, J. C., Lewy, A. J., Goodwin, F. K., Davenport, Y., Mueller, P. S., Newsome, D. A., and Uehr, T. A., (1984). Seasonal affective disorder. *Archives of General Psychiatry, 41*, 72–80.

Rusak, B., & Zucker, I. (1975). Biological rhythms and animal behavior. *Annual Review of Psychology, 26*, 137–171.

Stephan, F. K., & Zucker, I. (1972). Circadian rhythms in drinking behavior and locomotor activity of rats are eliminated by hypothalamic lesions. *Proceedings of the National Academy of Sciences, USA, 69*, 1583–1586.

Weitzman, E. D., Czeisler, C. A., Coleman, R. M., Spielman, A. J., Zimmerman, J. C., & Dement, W. C. (1981). Delayed sleep phase syndrome: A chronobiological disorder with sleep onset insomnia. *Archives of General Psychiatry, 38*, 737–746.

Part Five

Specific Populations

Unfortunately, insomnia is rarely the only symptom in our patients. In Chapter 14, Merrill Mitler and colleagues discuss the treatment of insomnia in patients with chronic medical illness. Pain, fever, pruritus, paresthesias, and coughing are some of the common symptoms that cause insomnia in the chronically ill. Mitler *et al.* advise the judicious use of sedative hypnotics, combined with wise scheduling of sleep-disrupting medications. Other cases are best treated by tricyclic antidepressants. According to Mitler *et al.*, the sleep disorders specialist must be knowledgeable about the realities of chronic medical illness and must be sensitive to the frustrations of both the patient and the internist.

The book closes with a chapter on treating sleep disturbances in the elderly, who are at a higher risk than younger adults both for sleep problems and for serious side effects from hypnotics. Behavioral treatments remain effective in this age group. However, it is also important to keep in mind the particular life-cycle issues that face older adults. One needs to determine whether an elderly person's insomnia has been precipitated by recent events (retirement, illness, death of a loved one) or whether it is related to unresolved issues of a previous life stage. Although relaxation training, stimulus control, sleep curtailment, and sleep hygiene are quite effective in the elderly, direct attention to developmental issues may be a particularly important adjunct to behavioral therapy in this group.

CHAPTER 14

Insomnia in the Chronically Ill

MERRILL M. MITLER, STEVEN POCETA, STUART J. MENN, AND MILTON K. ERMAN

INTRODUCTION

Many patients with chronic diseases have insomnia stemming either directly from the symptoms of their illnesses or secondarily from procedures and medications used to treat their illnesses. Pain, fever, pruritus, paresthesias, diarrhea, and coughing are some of the common symptoms that cause insomnia in the chronically ill. Disrupted sleep–wake cycles due to therapeutic maneuvers and administration of medications are common iatrogenic factors leading to insomnia. Furthermore, underlying medical conditions may be exacerbated by sleep, by certain stages of sleep, or by sleeping in the recumbent position, thus contributing to sleep disruption. Furthermore, all insomnias can be complicated by and/or propagated by conditioning factors, even after the primary causes have abated.

This chapter deals with rational ways to manage complaints of insomnia seen in association with chronic illness or disease. We first present in detail several specific, common examples of such insomnias. Then we discuss how many of the therapeutic principles we employ are applicable to other forms of insomnia associated with chronic illness.

Disease-related insomnia is ubiquitous in our society. And, because increasing age is associated with increasing probability of disease, the

---

Merrill M. Mitler, Steven Poceta, Stuart J. Menn, and Milton K. Erman • Sleep Disorders Center, Scripps Clinic and Research Foundation, La Jolla, California 92037.

prevalence of disease-related insomnia is expected to grow apace with the mean age of our population.

Insomnia is one of the five complaints voiced most often by patients with chronic respiratory diseases (Prigatano, Wright, & Levin, 1984; Cattarall, Douglas, Calverley, Brash, Brezinova, Shapiro, & Flenley, 1982; Timms, Dawson, Hajdukovic, & Mitler, 1988). For example, a typical night for a stable patient with even mild chronic obstructive pulmonary disease (COPD) is characterized by sleep disturbances associated with the need to clear secretions in the respiratory tract or to wake up for administration of medications. Moreover, COPD patients experience pharmacologically based sleep disruptions from respiratory stimulants (e.g., theophylline) and perhaps steroids (Mandell, Walker, Steinherz, & Fuks, 1989; Webb, 1981).

Other common chronic medical conditions with disruptive effects on sleep include congestive heart failure, rheumatic pain conditions, and neurologic diseases. Patients with chronic heart failure often have a sleep disturbance associated with Cheyne–Stokes respiration or paroxysmal nocturnal dyspnea (Rees & Clark, 1979; Anch, Browman, Mitler, & Walsh, 1988). Over 30 years ago, the sleep disruption of migraine headache was well recognized (Gans, 1954). The insomnia-producing effects of restless-legs syndrome and nocturnal myoclonus are also well described (Ekbom, 1945; Association of Sleep Disorders Centers, 1979; Coleman, Bliwise, Sajben, de Bruyn, Boomkamp, Menn, & Dement, 1983). The dysesthesia of diabetic polyneuropathy is classically nocturnal. Fibromyalgia and other rheumatic conditions associated with chronic pain are also associated with the complaint of insomnia and alpha frequency intrusions in the sleep electroencephalogram (EEG) (Smythe & Moldofsky, 1977; Moldofsky, Lue, & Smythe, 1979; Hench & Mitler, 1986a,b). Virtually all patients with Parkinson's disease have some form of insomnia, which is related to the specific neurodegenerative state and to nonspecific factors, such as the immobility produced when L-DOPA wears off (Klawans, Carvey, Tanner, & Goetz, 1986).

METHOD

Our approach to the complaint of insomnia in the chronically ill is the same as that for any symptom—a thorough history and physical examination are completed and appropriate laboratory data are gathered. A differential diagnostic tree is created. We consider that all insomnia can be due to one or more of the following:

1. Medical illness (e.g., hyperthyroidism)
2. Symptoms of medical illness (e.g., pain)

3. Primary sleep disorder (e.g., sleep apnea or nocturnal myoclonus)
4. Psychiatric illness (e.g., depression)
5. Psychophysiological conditioning

If the history, physical examination, and screening laboratory data do not clearly favor one specific diagnosis, then an overnight sleep recording may be necessary before a specific treatment regimen is begun.

If a specific chronic illness is judged to be a major factor causing insomnia, a goal of the treatment is to help the patient and the primary-care physician appreciate the complex interrelationships among the patient's medical condition, sleep physiology, and current treatment plan. Achieving this goal may require one or more patient visits after an initial consultation and a thorough discussion with the primary-care physician. Key features to explore are discussed next.

Effect of the Primary Disease on Sleep

Those involved with caring for a COPD patient should be aware of the effect of increased airways resistance on sleep and the effect of the paralysis of accessory breathing muscles during rapid-eye-movement (REM) sleep on respiration. All involved with the care of an arthritic patient should realize the relationship between restricted or painful movements during the night and disrupted sleep. Table 1 lists several common conditions that can adversely affect sleep patterns.

Effect of Therapeutic Intervention on Sleep

The most common example of this effect may be the impact on sleep physiology and on the wake–sleep cycle of respiratory stimulant medications (e.g., xanthines—caffeine-like drugs including theophylline) and therapeutic maneuvers during the night (e.g., movements and activities to clear the airways). If alerting medications must be given, their use should be avoided after 6:00 P.M. All necessary therapeutic maneuvers should be performed in dim light. Other procedures (e.g., vital signs, neurologic assessment, etc.) should be performed in a manner that minimizes disruption of the wakefulness–sleep cycle. Certain medications can adversely affect sleep quality whenever they are given; some of these are listed in Table 2. Sometimes, a change from one medication to another of the same class can be helpful.

Patient Control over Sleep

Regular, nightly use of sedatives may be quite appropriate for patients with terminal illnesses and for some patients with chronic illnesses.

Table 1. Medical Conditions Associated with Insomnia

Central nervous system conditions
    Mass lesion (e.g., hypothalamic tumor, increased intracranial pressure)
    Vascular headache (e.g., cluster headache, migraine)
    Infection (e.g., encephalitis)
    Degenerative conditions (e.g., Alzheimer's disease, Parkinson's disease)
    Trauma
    Toxic encephalopathy or withdrawal states
    Epilepsy (e.g., nocturnal seizures or medications)
    Muscle and peripheral nerve disorders (e.g., diabetic neuropathy, amyotrophic lateral sclerosis, myotonic dystrophy)
Other medical problems
    Endocrine and metabolic diseases (e.g., hyperthyroidism)
    Renal failure (e.g., postdialysis disequilibirium syndrome)
    Hepatic failure (e.g., nocturnal delirium)
    Infection (e.g., pyrexia or night sweats)
    Rheumatologic disorders (e.g., fibromyalgia)
    Gastrointestinal disorders (e.g., gastroesophageal reflux, inflammatory bowel disease)
    Alcohol abuse
    Asthma
    Obstructive or restrictive pulmonary disease
    Congestive heart failure
    Prolonged, unavoidable time in bed for any reason

Furthermore, intermittent use of sedatives in stable, chronically ill patients can give them a real sense of control over their insomnia. Behavioral strategies for treating and coping with insomnia are as important in medically based insomnia as in psychophysiological insomnia. Often, to feel better, patients must simply understand that some nights will be poor, but others will be better, and that they will not suffer significant physical harm from the sleepless nights (Table 3).

Treatment of medically based insomnia must include sleep hygiene and reinforcement of the basic 24-hour wakefulness–sleep pattern. Unfortunately, many patients (e.g., poststroke) cannot follow the typical stimulus-control treatment regimen of getting out of bed when not asleep. Nonetheless, for the majority of patients, proper sleep hygiene and planned activities if sleepless are the cornerstones of treatment. When physical illness interferes with mobility, regular morning activities and the use of scheduled bright-light therapy can be helpful. Exposure to light must be minimized during the usual sleeping hours even if the patient is unable to sleep. Depression is common in the chronically ill and should be treated if present.

The use of benzodiazepine hypnotics is appropriate for certain pa-

Table 2. Common Medications that May Cause Insomnia

Corticosteroids
Beta blockers
Respiratory stimulants (e.g., theophylline, metaproterenol)
Immunosupression (e.g., methotrexate, cyclosporine)
Phenytoin
Monoamine oxidase inhibitors
Methyldopa (Aldomet)
Caffeine (Excedrin/Fiorinal/Cafergot)
Alerting antidepressants [Vivactil (protriptyline), Prozac (fluoxetine), Wellbutrin (buproprion), etc.]
Illicit, recreational drugs (stimulating drugs during their use and sedating drugs during their discontinuation)
Alcohol use

tients. We use them in pain syndromes, movement disorders, states of impaired mobility (bed-bound patients), and severe chronic insomnia not treatable by other measures, such as the insomnia of chronic (abstinent) former alcoholics. We avoid benzodiazepines in patients who tend to escalate the amount of drug taken for sleep or to otherwise abuse drugs, persons with impaired cognition or coordination who must walk to the bathroom at night, and in those with significant respiratory impairments (but see below). The duration of use must be dictated by the clinical circumstances. Ideally, the patient will use the drug only intermittently, such as after several poor nights of sleep. We discourage use in the middle of the night and instead attempt to decrease the patient's fear of and reaction to insomnia. A "planned" sedative, taken at bedtime, is preferable. If the condition causing the insomnia is chronic and not amenable to other treatments, regular use of a benzodiazepine can be recommended. We discourage nightly use, but have had good experience with a flexible every-other-night regimen (averaging three or four drug nights per week)

Table 3. Stategies for Control of Insomnia in the Chronically Ill Patient

Optimize medical condition
Patient acceptance and understanding of insomnia
Daytime naps
Intermittent use of sedatives
Frequent visits to physician
Nonpharmacological treatments (e.g., sleep hygiene, sleep restriction, relaxation techniques, biofeedback, hypnosis)

in patients with periodic leg movements and patients with fibromyalgia (Mitler, Browman, Menn, Gujavarty, & Timms, 1986; Hench & Mitler, 1986a,b). We doubt that rebound insomnia occurs when dosing is every other night. Some patients may prefer to use a hypnotic nightly for up to a month and then taper off and discontinue its use for a period of days or weeks. Our rationale for choosing an intermittent medication regime is as follows: (1) Available sleep laboratory studies and our own clinical experience indicate that the commonly used benzodiazepines probably do not provide efficacy beyond four to five weeks of nightly use. (2) Our clinical experience is that chronic nightly use of sedative benzodiazepines is often associated with dependence. (3) We have seen no clinical evidence of loss of efficacy over years with use three or four nights per week.

For example, insomnia in stable, non-CO_2-retaining COPD patients with mild to moderate disease responds well to 0.125 to 0.25 mg of triazolam at bedtime (Timms, Dawson, Hajdukovic, & Mitler, 1988). Even though it is necessary to stop this type of sedation during intervals of disease exacerbation, when there may be CO_2 retention or other acute respiratory problems, and even though sleep continues to be poor on nondrug nights, our COPD patients find that with prolonged intermittent use they gain a sense of control over their chronic sleep disturbances. We also have seen good clinical responses with the intermittent use of sedative benzodiazepines (e.g., temazepam or triazolam) in the pain and sleep disturbance of fibromyalgia (Hench, Cohen, & Mitler, 1989).

Sedating tricyclic antidepressants are useful in cases where pain is a major aspect of the insomnia. These medications, particularly amitriptyline, doxepin, and imipramine, are now used to treat neuropathic pain, such as diabetic neuropathy, musculoskeletal pain, tension and vascular headaches, and psychiatric disorders, such as pain disorder, anxiety, and depression. Also, we often use them to treat insomnia associated with respiratory compromise. For some patients (e.g., those with asthma), the anticholinergic effects are welcome, but for others (e.g., those with confusion and urinary hesitancy), these effects significantly limit their use. There are advantages and drawbacks to persistent use of any sedative, and they must be administered in combination with patient education. Certainly, an educated doctor's prescription seems preferable to self-treatment with alcohol or over-the-counter sleep aids.

CASE 1: HYPNOGENIC DYSTONIA

A 36-year-old man presented to the Rheumatology Division at Scripps Clinic because of complaints of back spasms occurring at night leading to sleep disruption and daytime sleepiness. These spasms involved the low back and seemed to be related to a lifting injury the patient had suffered a few months earlier. Treatment with conservative measures and nonsteroidal anti-inflammatory agents was only partly successful. Diazepam finally produced relief from these spasms, which were occurring as often as 10 to 12 times per night. Unfortunately, doses as high as 15 mg were needed to control the spasms, and the patient was experiencing significant daytime sedation as a result. He was referred for neurologic and sleep evaluations.

Further history revealed that the spasms and insomnia had begun gradually, and that the patient had no sleeping partner. Once, however, when on vacation at a friend's house, his host commented on the restlessness and noise that the patient made at night, of which he was unaware. Additionally, the patient related two episodes in which he was awakened from sleep by back spasms, but immediately felt himself losing vision and consciousness, waking up sometime later. There was never a history of urinary or fecal incontinence or of tongue biting. The physical examination was completely normal, and imaging studies of the head and spine showed no abnormalities except a grade 1 lumbar spondylolysis. The routine EEG was normal.

Overnight polysomnography with 16-channel EEG, performed with the patient off diazepam, demonstrated two spells occurring directly out of stage 2 sleep in which the patient flexed his legs up into a "frog-leg" position, awoke, and had strong rhythmic contractions of the lower extremities. No EEG abnormalities were seen, and a diagnosis of paroxysmal nocturnal dystonia was made (Cirignotta, Lugaresi & Montagna, 1989). Treatment with carbamazepine was instituted, and the patient has not had further episodes (except when he tapered the medication) and has not had daytime drowsiness.

This case demonstrates the need for proper diagnosis of conditions that can present as insomnia. The patient was initially thought to have insomnia due to a minor injury causing lower back pain, but more detailed evaluation revealed a specific parasomnia condition which responded well to specific and appropriate treatment.

CASE 2: INSOMNIA SECONDARY TO CARDIOGENIC NOCTURNAL DYSPNEA

Mr. BH, a 66-year-old man with severe ischemic cardiomyopathy and repetitive paroxysmal nocturnal dyspnea and orthopnea, was hospitalized for evaluation and treatment of his dyspnea and secondary insomnia.

Sleep apnea screening studies were performed on three consecutive nights of his hospitalization. These consisted of continuous monitoring with a pulse oximeter and respiratory strain gauges over a minimum of 7.5 hours each night, producing a continuous recording of arterial saturation and respiratory excursion. The procedures were performed while the patient was breathing room air. The records were analyzed for mean arterial saturation, minimum arterial saturation, number of desaturation events, type (central or obstructive), and frequency of apneas. On the first night of monitoring, the patient took his usual cardiac medications (digoxin, 0.375 mg daily, and furosemide, 160 mg three times a day). To simulate his habitual alcohol consumption patterns, he was allowed to drink 4 ounces of whiskey before bed. On the second night, he took his usual medications without whiskey or other sedatives. On the third night, he took his usual medications plus medroxyprogesterone (10 mg three times a day) and theophylline (200 mg twice a day).

On all three nights, the oxygenation and respiration records revealed 150 to 200 apneas, each preceded by gradual decreases and followed by gradual increases in respiratory effort. These events were episodic and presumably related to sleep. The patient had a mean arterial saturation of 93 percent and a minimum of 81 percent. There were no clinically significant changes from night to night in his objective sleep parameters. He showed no significant change on the third night after the therapeutic interventions with theophylline and progesterone and no effect from discontinuation of alcohol. However, he reported that his sleep had improved on his third study night. A diagnosis was made of Cheyne–Stokes respiration (periodic breathing due to increased circulation time of the blood) secondary to cardiomyopathy. The respiratory abnormality was felt to cause his insomnia. There was no significant contribution to the insomnia from true congestive heart failure or pulmonary edema, but the insomnia was complicated by alcohol use. Although full polysomnography could not be performed, the periodic breathing pattern and subsequent movements (arousals) were obvious and felt to be diagnostic of this disorder.

Mr. BH was discharged on lower doses of digoxin and furosemide. Theophylline and medroxyprogesterone were added as respiratory stimulants. He experienced no improvement in sleep. Amitriptyline was therefore begun at an initial dose of 100 mg and gradually increased in 10-mg increments to a final dose of 50 mg. Subjective reports from the patient and his wife were that the amitriptyline produced a dramatic improvement in sleep. The patient's wife reported that some four weeks after amitriptyline was initiated, his sleep became less restful and characterized by some episodes of respiratory irregularity, which may have been apnea. However, he remained lively and mentally active during the day and took no daytime naps. On the whole, he felt better. His only complaint was of possible slight enlargement of the left groin with a pulsatile mass, an area where he previously had an arterial graft. He also complained of weakness, but otherwise presented with no specific cardiovascular problems.

Our impression was that the patient's cardiomyopathy was close to being optimally treated and that the sleep disruption was secondary to sleep apnea. We felt that the apnea was subjectively improved by amitriptyline, but may still have been undertreated. We planned to follow the patient medically, to increase amitriptyline to 75 mg at bedtime, and to reevaluate respiration during sleep in three months.

On a subsequent admission three months later, Mr. BH underwent follow-up study of nocturnal oxygenation and respiration in connection with his wife's observations of sleep apnea and relief of subjective sleep disruption by amitriptyline. This study showed the same recurrent sleep apneas (Cheyne–Stokes type) as did the previous studies (when he was severely symptomatic). The only change noted on amitriptyline appeared to be less arousal with the postapneic breathing.

The patient developed malaise and weakness. Despite vigorous amiloride and potassium therapy, hypokalemia was present, which was later corrected. The diuretics were further reduced. There was no significant ventricular ectopy. The patient developed atrial fibrillation and remained in fibrillation until the day of discharge. Hospitalization was otherwise unremarkable. Hemodynamics were satisfactorily controlled with the help of pulmonary artery monitoring, and there were no hemodynamic complications. The patient was discharged to outpatient follow-up with the intent to continue aggressive treatment of his cardiomyopathy. Theophylline, progesterone, and amitriptyline were continued for respiratory stimulation and sedation. These measures helped, but we were unable to completely eliminate the periodic breathing and resultant sleep disruption.

This case exemplifies the clinical experience at Scripps Clinic that proper treatment of patients with insomnia associated with congestive heart failure can produce symptomatic improvement with better sleep at night. Such patients rarely do well on benzodiazepines. We have found it necessary to decide whether the nocturnal breathing disturbance is related to paroxysmal nocturnal dyspnea and pulmonary edema or to low cardiac output and Cheyne–Stokes respirations with associated agitation and restlessness. When pulmonary edema is involved, increased diuresis may make the patient more comfortable at night, but this has no effect if the primary disturbance is a form of central sleep apnea and the patient is already well compensated. Additionally, amitriptyline or imipramine may be effective sedatives without the risk of respiratory depression.

These cases are very difficult to treat, and at times only minimal subjective improvement is achieved. In some medical conditions, the associated insomnia may be essentially incurable. For example, one patient with inflammatory bowel (Crohn's) disease reports that her jejunostomy bag fills up every two hours and irritates the skin if she is supine. Another patient who has had a stroke has no one at home to get her out of bed between 8:00 P.M. and 8:00 A.M., leading to a prolonged time in bed and low sleep efficiency. The sleep disorders specialist must be sensitive to the realities of chronic medical illness as well as to the frustration of the patient and internist. Only after these realities and frustrations are appreciated can goals for the improvement of sleep be set appropriately.

DISCUSSION

Our approach may be considered an aggressive extension of the medical model used by most sleep disorders centers. However, in our program, we actively encourage referral of patients with chronic illnesses because we feel that sleep is often an ignored facet of their overall management. Consider several brief examples of how our approach can be applied.

> A 68-year-old man with rheumatoid arthritis has been put on a steroid medication to reduce pain and swelling. Since he started taking the drug, he has complained of insomnia.

Many drugs (e.g., see Table 2), even when properly used, can have disruptive effects on sleep. The best approach to insomnia caused by the use of a needed medication is to adjust the time of the day that the drug is taken and the dose of the medication in hopes of keeping the therapeutic effect and reducing the side effect. Another possibility is to have the treating physician prescribe a different drug in the same class of medications. Often, the treatment is temporary and may be given in conjunction with a sedative benzodiazepine at bedtime. There are no good studies regarding the optimal treatment of sleep-disrupting drugs. For example, there is ample clinical experience that steroids disrupt sleep. However, there are no objective studies on dose response or duration of action. There is also no objective information on the relationship between steroid-induced insomnia and steriod-induced psychosis. However, we have successfully used lithium carbonate in conjunction with steroid-induced mania and sleeplessness (Falk, 1981), and clonazepam may also offer some hope in this situation (Viswanathan & Glickman, 1989). Finally, there is no data in the literature or in clinical practice on the effect of nonsteroidal anti-inflammatory agents on sleep. In fact, drowsiness is sometimes listed as a rare central side effect. While nonsteroidals are rarely good substitutes for steroids, the lack of sleep disruption does represent an important reason to consider using a nonsteroidal drug when chronic anti-inflammatory action is required.

> A 53-year-old woman has asthma with breathing difficulty mainly during the day. Recently, however, she was hospitalized two times in one month for asthma attacks during the night. This disrupted not only her sleep, but that of the entire household.

Asthmatic attacks can be triggered by allergic and/or emotional reactions. While exclusively sleep-related attacks are somewhat rare, it is not uncommon for some asthmatics to have a greater problem during the night. Daytime attacks can often be avoided or self-treated with inhaled medications. One of the main reasons asthma may "break through" during sleep is that the therapeutic effects of anti-asthmatic medications taken during the waking hours may not last throughout the sleeping hours. However, there are several other reasons why sleep may be directly involved in bringing on asthmatic attacks: (1) Sleep is associated with a mild increase in airway resistance in the normal person, and this change may play a role in some asthmatic attacks during sleep. (2) During REM sleep, there are profound changes in autonomic nervous system function which can affect heart and lung activity, especially in producing cardiac irregularities. These physiological changes could trigger asthmatic attacks. (3) Sleep-related esophageal reflux, which occurs to some extent in all people, can apparently cause bronchospasm in some asthmatic patients. (4) Finally, during sleep, asthmatics may not be able to self-medicate as quickly after the first signs of an attack as they can during wakefulness.

> A 65-year-old man presents complaining of burning leg pain, which is most troublesome during the night and most severe in the feet. A medical workup reveals mild diabetes with an associated polyneuropathy.

Neuropathic pain of many kinds can be most severe at night, but pain of any origin—the most common might be low back strain—can keep people awake. Depending on the chronicity of the problem and the patient's drug-taking habits, the underlying problem should usually be treated directly. Amitriptyline (and certain other tricyclic compounds) is an excellent treatment for the pain of neuropathies, and the sedative effect is often welcome. Treatment of acute low back pain might be accomplished with codeine, thus improving sleep, whereas the early morning back and leg pain of Parkinson's disease would be better treated with a midnight dose of L-DOPA or perhaps imipramine at bedtime. Treatment of the chronic pain of fibromyalgia is problematic. Moldofsky (1989) has suggested that fibromyalgia is best treated with a tripartite approach involving a sedating antidepressant, such as amitriptyline, moderate exercise, and supportive psychotherapy, and we agree with this clinical approach. From a research point of view, we are currently comparing the efficacy of amitriptyline with that of sedative benzodiazepines (temazepam, triazolam, and clonazepam). Our preliminary results (Hench, Cohen, & Mitler, 1989) indicate that there is no significant difference between amitriptyline and temazepam in terms of their effects on the clinical or sleep laboratory measures in fibromyalgia.

Merrill M. Mitler received his Ph.D. in Psychology from Michigan State University in 1970. Dr. Mitler did postdoctoral training in sleep physiology and sleep disorders at Stanford University School of Medicine from 1970 to 1973. He served under William Dement as Administrative Director of Stanford's Sleep Disorders Center from 1977 to 1978. In 1978, Dr. Mitler founded and directed the SUNY— Stony Brook Sleep Disorders Center. In 1983, Dr. Mitler moved to Scripps Clinic and Research Foundation in La Jolla, California, where he serves as Member (Professor) at the Research Institute and as Director of Research for the Division of Sleep Disorders. Dr. Mitler served for 12 years as Executive Secretary-Treasurer of the Association of Sleep Disorders Centers (now known as the American Sleep Disorders Association) and has authored two books and over 200 scientific articles. In 1984, Dr. Mitler was awarded the Nathaniel Kleitman Award by the American Sleep Disorders Association. Dr. Mitler is a member of the Board of Directors of the American Narcolepsy Association.

Steven Poceta received his M.D. from the University of Pennsylvania in 1983. He completed his residency in Neurology at the University of Washington in 1987 and did a Fellowship in Sleep Medicine at Scripps Clinic in 1988. He joined the faculty of the Scripps Clinic Sleep Disorders Center in 1988.

Stuart J. Menn received his M.D. from New York University in 1964. In 1969, he completed his residency in Medicine at The University of Vermont. He was a Fellow in the Department of Anesthesia at Harvard Medical School from 1969 to 1970 and a Fellow in Pulmonary Medicine at the University of California, San Diego, from 1970 to 1972. His interest in sleep disorders dates to the early 1970s when he did some of the first recordings on patients with sleep apnea in San Diego. He was cofounder of the Scripps Clinic Sleep Disorders Center in 1982. Dr. Menn serves on the Diagnostic Classification Committee of the American Sleep Disorders Association.

Milton K. Erman received his M.D. degree from 1975 at New York University. Dr. Erman did his residency in Psychiatry at the Massachusetts General Hospital between 1975 and 1978 and completed a fellowship in Consultation–Liaison Psychiatry at the Massachusetts General Hospital in 1978–1979. Dr. Erman was on the faculty of the University of Texas Health Sciences Center at Dallas from 1979 to

1986, serving as Associate Professor of Psychiatry. Working with Dr. Howard Roffwarg, he developed the University's Sleep Disorders Center at Presbyterian Hospital of Dallas and served as its Director prior to his move to Scripps Clinic in 1986. He is currently Head of the Division of Sleep Disorders at Scripps Clinic and Research Foundation and Director of its Sleep Disorders Center. Dr. Erman is the author of over 70 articles on the diagnosis and management of sleep disorders. He has served on the Accreditation Board of the American Sleep Disorders Association.

RECOMMENDED READINGS

Gillin, J. C., & Byerley, W. F. (1990), The diagnosis and management of insomnia, *New England Journal of Medicine, 332,* 239–248.
This is an excellent overview of symptoms and management for the doctoral-level professional.

Mitler, E. A., & Mitler, M. M. (1988). *101 questions about sleep and dreams* (2nd ed.). Del Mar, CA: Wakefulness–Sleep Education and Research Foundation.
This brief question-and-answer booklet provides a good orientation to sleep and sleep pathology for patients and ancillary personnel.

Mitler, M. M., and Erman, M. K. (Eds.) (in preparation). *The complaint of insomnia in the practice of medicine.* New York: Raven Press.
Proceedings of a symposium in which authorities representing various medical subspecialties (e.g., cardiology, neurology, pulmonology, rheumatology, and psychiatry) review the diagnosis and management of insomnia in their practices.

REFERENCES

Anch, A. M., Browman, C. P., Mitler, M. M., & Walsh, J. K. (1988). *Sleep: A scientific perspective.* Englewood Cliffs, NJ: Prentice-Hall, pp. 163–166.

Association of Sleep Disorders Centers, Sleep Disorders Classification Committee (Roffwarg, H. P., Chairman). (1979). Diagnostic classification of sleep and arousal disorders (1st ed.). *Sleep, 2,* 1–137.

Cattarall, J. R., Douglas, N. J., Calverley, P. M., Brash, H. M., Brezinova, V., Shapiro, C. M., & Flenley, D. C. (1982). Irregular breathing and hypoxaemia during sleep in chronic stable asthma. *Lancet, 1,* 301–304.

Cirignotta, F., Lugaresi, E., & Montagna, P. (1989). Nocturnal paroxysmal dystonia. In M. H. Kryger, T. Roth, & W. C. Dement (Eds.), *Principles and practice of sleep medicine.* New York: W. B. Saunders, pp. 410–412.

Coleman, R. M., Bliwise, D. L., Sajben, N., de Bruyn, L. Boomkamp, A., Menn, M. E., & Dement, W. C. (1983). Epidemiology of periodic movements during sleep. In C. Guilleminault & E. Lugaresi (Eds.), *Sleep/wake disorders: Natural history, epidemiology and long term evolution.* New York, Raven Press, pp. 217–229.

Ekbom, K. A. (1945). Restless legs. *Acta Medica Scandinavica, 158* (Suppl.) 1–123.

Falk, W. E. (1981). Steroid psychosis: Diagnosis and treatment. In T. C. Manschreck (Ed.), *Psychiatric medicine update*. New York: Elsevier, pp. 147–154.

Gans, M. (1954). Migraine is a form of neurasthenia. *Journal of Nervous and Mental Diseases, 113*, 315–331.

Hench, P. K., Cohen, R., & Mitler, M. M. (1989). Fibromyalgia: Effects of temazepam, amitriptyline and placebo on pain and sleep. *Sleep Research, 18*, 335.

Hench, P. K., & Mitler, M. M. (1986a). Fibromyalgia 1. Review of a common rheumatologic syndrome. *Postgraduate Medicine, 80*, 47–56.

Hench, P. K., & Mitler M. M. (1986b). Fibromyalgia 2. Management guidelines and research findings. *Postgraduate Medicine, 80*, 57–69.

Klawans, H. L., Carvey, P. M., Tanner, C. M., & Goetz, C. G. (1986). Drug-induced myoclonus. In S. Fahn, C. D. Marsden, & M. H. van Woert (Eds.), *Myoclonus. Advances in neurology* (Vol. 43). New York: Raven Press, pp. 251–264.

Mandell, L. R., Walker, R. W., Steinherz, P., & Fuks, Z. (1989). Reduced incidence of the somnolence syndrome in leukemic children with steroid coverage during prophylactic cranial radiation therapy. Results of a pilot study. *Cancer, 63*, 1975–1978.

Mitler, M. M., Browman, C. P., Menn, S. J., Gujavarty, K., & Timms, R. M. (1986). Nocturnal myoclonus: Treatment efficacy of clonazepam and temazepam. *Sleep, 9*, 385–392.

Moldofsky, H. (1989). Sleep and fibrositis syndrome. *Rheumatic Diseases Clinics of North America, 15*(1), 91–103.

Moldofsky, H., Lue, F., & Smythe, H. (1979). Alpha EEG sleep and pain in rheumatoid arthritis. *Sleep Research, 8*, 236.

Prigatano, G. P., Wright, E. C., & Levin, D. (1984). Quality of life and its predictors in patients with mild hypoxemia and chronic obstructive pulmonary disease. *Archives of Internal Medicine, 144*, 1613–1619.

Rees, P. J., & Clark, T. J. (1979). Paroxysmal nocturnal dyspnoea and periodic respiration. *Lancet, 2*(8156–8157), 1315–1317.

Smythe, H. A., & Moldofsky, H. (1977). Two contributions to the understanding of the fibrositis syndrome. *Bulletin of the Rheumatic Diseases, 28*, 928–931.

Timms, R. M., Dawson, A., Hajdukovic, R. M., & Mitler, M. M. (1988). Effect of triazolam on sleep and arterial oxygen saturation in patients with chronic obstructive pulmonary disease. *Archives of Internal Medicine, 148*, 2159–2163.

Viswanathan, R. L., & Glickman, L. (1989). Clonazepam in the treatment of steroid-induced mania in a patient after renal transplantation. *New England Journal of Medicine, 320*, 319–320.

Webb, D. R. (1981). Steroids in allergic disease. *Medical Clinics of North America, 65*, 1073–1081.

CHAPTER FIFTEEN

Insomnia in the Older Adult

JUDITH FLAXMAN

INTRODUCTION

Nearly half the adults between the ages of 65 and 79 (45 percent) report some difficulty with insomnia (Bootzin & Engle-Friedman, 1987). Additionally, nearly half of 65-to-74-year-olds use hypnotics regularly (Rosenberg, 1984). This percentage is even higher for the institutionalized elderly. This high use of hypnotics is a serious problem for older adults because they often use multiple medications and do not metabolize drugs efficiently.

The statistics on sleep problems in older adults show that increased wakefulness and decreased slow-wave sleep are two major effects of aging. Although these changes may be subjectively experienced as less sound sleep, they do not create problems for all older adults (Prinz & Raskind, 1978).

Few treatment studies have focused exclusively on the sleep problems of older adults. One controlled outcome study (Bootzin & Engle-Friedman, 1987) successfully treated individuals between the ages of 47 and 76 using various combinations of support, sleep hygiene information, progressive relaxation training, and stimulus control instructions. This study showed that it was even possible to reverse some of the most highly age-associated trends in sleep—night-time awakenings and nap taking. A recent multiple case study (Hoelscher & Edinger, 1988) used sleep period restriction, sleep education, and stimulus control instructions to successfully treat four of five older adult subjects who had sleep-maintenance insomnia.

Judith Flaxman • Illinois School of Professional Psychology, Chicago, Illinois 60604.

Despite age-related changes in sleep characteristics, older insomniacs' sleep is not qualitatively different from younger insomniacs' sleep (i.e., the sleep of young and old insomniacs differs in similar ways from that of normal sleepers; Bootzin & Engle-Friedman, 1987). It is, thus, reasonable to expect that treatment approaches developed for the general adult population will work for the older adult population as well.

Older insomniacs are likely to be dealing with different life issues than younger insomniacs. Issues such as understanding one's own aging, death and dying, and coping with chronic illness and disability are important for this population (Knight, 1986). For some clients the stress that these life cycle issues can create must be addressed in treatment, rather than other issues that are more common in a younger population.

METHOD

A client is referred to me from an accredited sleep disorders center where he or she has already had a physical and neurological examination and, in some cases, a polysomnographic examination, if the examining neurologist and polysomnographer believe the latter to be warranted. This referral route ensures that individuals with sleep apnea or periodic leg movements ("restless legs" syndrome) are screened out, or provided with medical treatment, before they reach me. Since the incidence of these problems is higher in the older adult population, this is an important safeguard.

I conduct a clinical interview in order to identify the psychological factors that have resulted in and are maintaining the sleep problem. I find that an interview with the client (including a family member, if possible) is adequate for assessing these factors.

In my clinical interview, I search for the most important etiological factors and maintaining conditions. In doing this, I keep in mind the more common psychological factors involved, as listed in Table 1. I explore these with the client, as I work toward developing a conceptualization of the sleep problem that I can share with the client.

As I engage in this diagnostic process, I am aware that if the problem is chronic, or if life-cycle changes have occurred since the problem began, the factors that initiated the sleep disorder may not be currently maintaining it.

I develop an individualized treatment plan based on my assessment. I discuss this plan with the client and estimate how many sessions of treatment will be needed (typically about four sessions).

An outline of the various treatment possibilities is presented in Table

Table 1. *Etiological Factors, Current Conditions, and Treatment Approaches*

Etiology and current conditions	Treatment
Psychopathology	
Depression	Activity scheduling, cognitive restructuring
Generalized anxiety	Relaxation training, exercise, cognitive restructuring
Panic attacks	Relaxation training, paradoxical intention (Chambless, Goldstein, Gallagher, and Bright, 1986)
Personality style	
Obsessive	Thought stopping, worry time
Perfectionistic	Cognitive restructuring
Type A	Relaxation, Imagery
Life stress	
Work demands	Life-style balance (Marlatt, 1985), time management
Caretaker responsibilities	Life-style balance, time management
Life-cycle issues	
Retirement	Retirement counseling
Feelings about aging	Life review (Knight, 1986)
Death, dying, and grief	Grief counseling (Worden, 1982)
Sleep-related issues	
Conditioned insomnia	Stimulus control, sleep hygiene
Performance anxiety	Education, systematic desensitization
Secondary gain for sleep problem	Family or marital therapy

1. The treatment plan will almost invariably include standard sleep hygiene, stimulus control, and relaxation techniques. It may also include techniques aimed at dealing with depression, such as activity scheduling (Lewinsohn, Munoz, Youngren, & Zeiss, 1986) or cognitive restructuring (Beck, Rush, Shaw, & Emery, 1979). If a great deal of anxiety is present, thought stopping (Wolpe, 1969) as soon as a distressing thought begins, combined with engaging in an incompatible or distracting activity, relaxation as a coping skill (Goldfried & Trier, 1974), and other stress management techniques will be used. The latter include life-style balance (Marlatt, 1985), exercise (Martin & Dubbert, 1987), and time out for worry (Davis, Eshelman, & McKay, 1982).

Life-style balance (Marlatt, 1985) is the degree of equilibrium between daily activities that the individual perceives as external demands ("shoulds") and daily activities that the person engages in for pleasure or self-fulfillment ("wants"). An overabundance of "shoulds" is hypothesized to result in a perception of self-deprivation and a need for self-indulgence. I assume that it also creates stress and an inability to carry out new activities that could lead to improved sleep. I encourage some clients to record, or simply report, the balance between daily "wants" and "shoulds." We then plan activities to provide a better balance between the two.

Knight (1986) points out that older adults are often in need of various kinds of help, so other case work types of services are also provided, as needed. Bereavement work may be needed for individuals who are grieving over a loss. Other possible interventions are retirement counseling, to help the individual plan in a concrete way for the future, and "life review," which has variously been described as reminiscing about previous experiences to prepare for major developmental changes, as a search for meaning in life, or as the working through of unresolved conflicts from earlier developmental stages (Knight, 1986).

A SUCCESSFUL CASE

Mrs. E was a 59-year-old elementary-school teacher, one year away from retirement, who was experiencing sleep-maintenance insomnia. Mrs. E had been widowed nine years. For the previous two years she had been receiving psychotherapy on a weekly basis. Mrs. E's primary therapist described her as anxious and depressed.

Mrs. E's insomnia began three years earlier at a very stressful time in her life—she had become the confidante of a rather disturbed, alcoholic coworker, who later committed suicide; she was involved in an automobile accident that left her injured; and she had a particularly difficult class, which included two children who were eventually diagnosed as psychotic and were removed from the class quite late in the school year.

Mrs. E came to see me early in September, at the beginning of the school year. She was afraid that her insomnia would not allow her to function adequately in her job. She had coped with the sleep problem during the summer by napping when necessary, but she could not do this once school began.

With Mrs. E's permission, I consulted her primary therapist and we agreed on a division of labor. I would focus on the sleep problem and on techniques Mrs. E could use to control her anxiety and obsessive worrying. As much as possible, I would leave the actual content of the worries to Mrs. E's primary therapist. Mrs. E and I agreed to work together for three or four sessions.

Treatment

Mrs. E was given information aimed at reducing her performance anxiety concerning sleep. She was able to agree that she might not need as much sleep as she thought she did and that she had been able to function well despite being low on sleep. Additionally, she seemed to appreciate information about the high incidence of both sleep problems and frequent awakenings during the night. She enthusiastically shared this new information with her brother-in-law, who also had a sleep problem.

Sleep hygiene practices and stimulus control were reviewed and found to be adequate.

Relaxation training was carried out for Mrs. E using stretch relaxation (Carlson, Ventrella, & Sturgis, 1987), a variant of deep muscle relaxation I have found to be particularly effective for sleep disorders. I made an audio tape of the relaxation session I conducted in my office, which I gave to Mrs. E with instructions to use it nightly and record her level of tension before and after. I also scheduled a time when I would telephone Mrs. E, three days later, in order to "see how it's going" and find out whether or not she had any questions. This communicates the importance of the procedure to the client and allows the minor questions that often arise to be cleared up without losing a whole week (Stuart, 1980).

Several techniques were introduced to deal with Mrs. E's obsessive worrying. Thought stopping (Wolpe, 1969) was taught. A time out for worry (or worry time) was planned to occur an hour or so before bedtime (Davis, Eshelman, & McKay, 1982).

It is important to establish rules for the use of worry time. Mrs. E was instructed to review the events of the day and select one problem to focus on. She was to look for a solution (she saw herself as a "solution finder") but to remember that some problems cannot be solved in a day and that a solution would not always be in her power. I suggested that if she could not control the main problem, she should look for some aspect of it, or for something totally unrelated, that she could take control over (Maddi & Kobasa, 1984).

Mrs. E was told to use thought stopping and distraction once the worry time was over. Unresolved problems identified during the worry sessions were to be addressed with her primary therapist.

Mrs. E was able to use thought stopping and worry time to stop herself from obsessing over such issues as minor disagreements she had with colleagues during the day or the problems of her married daughter who lived in another part of the country.

Mrs. E was prone to take on too many responsibilities and lose sight of her priorities. This was becoming an increasing problem because she was approaching retirement and had not made plans for it. Since she felt she barely had time to carry out her job responsibilities (for example, carefully reworking old lesson plans), she was not able to make headway on planning for the future. I encouraged her to read a book on time management (Lakein, 1973). In the course of thinking about her priorities, Mrs. E was able to see more clearly that planning for retirement was important and that the lack of plans was creating stress for her. Working on this involved putting herself first. It also required that she decide that an old lesson plan was "good enough." She was able to make this shift.

As part of overcommitting herself and setting perfectionistic standards, Mrs. E did not allow herself to engage in any relaxing activities. This created stress for Mrs. E in the present and was also a problem for the future. Without enjoyable hobbies or a plan for her retirement, Mrs. E was quite worried about how she would spend her time. The idea of a balanced life style was introduced (Marlatt, 1985), and a list of enjoyable activities, including exercise, was developed, with guidelines for when and how to engage in these activities. For example, exercise was scheduled on a regular basis three times a week, and Friday nights were set aside for socializing or relaxing.

Results

Treatment resulted in the alleviation of Mrs. E's sleep-maintenance insomnia. A follow-up phone call to her ten months later found that Mrs. E had successfully used the techniques taught her. She had retired at the end of the school year and had terminated therapy with her primary therapist.

At the time of the follow-up call Mrs. E was having some trouble balancing various demands on her time. She was not allowing herself relaxation time in the evening. This was affecting her sleep, so that she generally awakened twice during the night. She was not distressed about this since she felt that she knew what to do to get the problem under control.

Discussion

In this case the problems that initiated the sleep problem were not the problems that maintained it. The stressful life events that contributed to the development of Mrs. E's sleep problem had been resolved by the time I saw her. The sleep problem had not, however, disappeared. Work on performance anxiety and on controlling Mrs. E's obsessive worrying and on developing a more balanced life-style solved the problem for approximately eight months. When the problem recurred because of a change in life-style due to Mrs. E's retirement, Mrs. E felt she had developed the skills to get it under control again.

AN UNSUCCESSFUL CASE

Mr. D was a 72-year-old business consultant working full-time. His sleep problems began when he was in his forties and involved both sleep-onset and sleep-maintenance insomnia. The problem had worsened in the past six months, and Mr. D's wife had urged him to seek treatment.

A number of life-cycle issues were affecting Mr. D. His only close friend had died suddenly two and a half years earlier. Mr. D himself had had a coronary bypass operation shortly afterward. Mr. D's wife had a mastectomy one year earlier. Mr. D observed that he had outlived his parents and older brother, all of whom had died in their sixties. He said that he felt that "they're calling our regiment." Additionally, Mr. D could not picture himself retiring. The idea distressed him greatly, although he felt he should slow down.

In addition to life-cycle problems, a number of life history problems existed as well. According to Mr. D, he and his wife barely communicated. Also, Mr. D was angry at, and felt used by, his son and daughter, whom he supported financially. He stated that in the past he had let them know how angry this made him, but at present he just put up with it.

Mr. D had many features of the type A personality (Friedman & Rosenman, 1974). He described himself as a person who got angry over little things (more in the past than in the present), was impatient with others, hard-driving, and "unable to turn off his motor." Affectively, Mr. D appeared depressed.

Treatment

I suggested relaxation training, time out for worry, and discussion of Mr. D's feelings about retirement as initial treatment approaches.

Mr. D was rather negative about all these suggestions. He was unwilling to go through a relaxation session, requesting instead that I explain the procedure to him so he could try it on his own at home. Lehrer (1982) has presented convincing evidence that it is quite important to actually carry out a relaxation session for the client. I was unable to persuade Mr. D of the value of this, however.

Mr. D stated that he did not need a time out for worry because he had no worries. He rejected the idea of discussing retirement, or anything else, on the grounds that talking does not solve problems.

Results

Mr. D went on a brief vacation after the assessment session and the single treatment session. He did not return to therapy as planned. A follow-up phone call about one month later found his sleep problem to be unchanged.

Discussion

Mr. D stated directly that he had come to therapy for a "gimmick." He seemed to view relaxation as such, but he was unwilling to give even that a real try. Mr. D was quite resistant about addressing difficult issues in his life.

It is interesting to contrast my failure with Mr. D with his (reportedly) successful participation in a cardiac rehabilitation program two years earlier. In reference to that program he said, "I'm a straightforward kind of guy. Just tell me what to do and I'll do it."

Several possibilities may explain why Mr. D reacted positively to one treatment program and negatively to another. One possibility is that the psychological nature of what I was asking Mr. D to do was quite threatening. Mr. D was quite resistant to talking about problems although he was open enough to acknowledge that the problems existed.

A second possibility is that Mr. D was unable to invest me, a therapist close to the ages of his children (viewed by him as "good-for-nothings"), with the necessary "referrent power" (Janis, 1983) for successful therapy to take place. The cardiologists running the cardiac rehabilitation program could more easily be viewed as trustworthy authority figures.

A third possibility is that Mr. D was benefitting in some way from his sleep problem. I did not have the opportunity to explore this, but I would have if Mr. D had returned to treatment. Mr. D did say that he sought treatment only because his wife urged him to do so. This tantalizing bit of information might be the key to a variety of different scenarios. Poor sleep may be rewarding for Mr. D because it is the way for him to get attention from his wife. Alternatively, Mr. D may be so hostile to his wife that he would deliberately fail to solve his sleep problem just to spite her.

Mr. D's case has many similarities to another case I treated at about the same time. Mr. S was also depressed, and he was also concerned about his retirement, his health, his wife's health, and issues of death and dying. Like Mr. D, he was also rather reluctant to discuss anything of a psychological nature. In contrast, to Mr. D, however, Mr. S appeared to have a very good marriage. His wife accompanied him to therapy and clearly showed her support for treatment. We used activity scheduling (Lewinsohn et al., 1986) to work on Mr. S's depression as he did not seem open to cognitive restructuring. Activity scheduling helped alleviate Mr. S's depression and also helped him develop interests he could pursue when he retired. We used sleep hygiene, relaxation, and stimulus control instructions for Mr. S's sleep problem. Treatment was quite successful.

DISCUSSION

I have had excellent success treating insomnia in the elderly using techniques demonstrated to be effective in younger insomniacs. It is important however, to tailor the treatment to the client's specific problems and to offer a wide variety of different techniques. In some cases, the specific techniques may be used as an adjunct to more standard therapy for life problems or to provide behavioral and less cognitive approaches for clients who are not psychologically minded.

At times it is difficult to overcome resistance due to marital problems, long-standing problems, or secondary gain. A special problem with the elderly may be resistance due to a generation gap between the client and therapist.

There are issues that are unique to the elderly and may need to be addressed in the treatment of insomnia. In many cases, these may not be the cause of the insomnia but may maintain the problem. These life-cycle problems include retirement, adjustment to loss of loved ones, and fear of death. Case work types of services may be helpful in dealing with these issues.

It is a mistake to assume that age-related changes in sleep necessarily result in insomnia and should, therefore, be tolerated by the elderly. Significant improvement in the quality of life can result from proper evaluation and treatment.

ACKNOWLEDGMENT

I thank Richard Rosenberg, Ph.D., for his helpful comments on an earlier draft of this chapter.

Judith Flaxman received her Ph.D. in Psychology from Northwestern University. She was an Assistant Professor of Psychology at the University of North Carolina at Chapel Hill and has been on the Core Faculty of the Illinois School of Professional Psychology since 1980. She is the Director of Psychological Services of the Multimodal Resource Center, a private outpatient mental health clinic. Dr. Flaxman has been a consultant for the Evanston Hospital Sleep Disorders Center since 1987.

RECOMMENDED READINGS

Davis, M., Eshelman, E. R., & McKay, M. (1982). *The relaxation and stress reduction workbook.* Oakland, CA: New Harbinger.
   An introductory workbook surveying popular relaxation and stress management techniques, appropriate for clients to read.
Knight, B. (1986). *Psychotherapy with older adults.* Beverly Hills, CA: Sage.
   Thoughtful coverage of all aspects of psychotherapy with older adults, including assessment. This book emphasizes a practical, behavioral approach but discusses other orientations to treatment as well.
Rosenberg, R. S. (1984). Aging and biological rhythms: Complaints of insomnia in the elderly. In E. Haus & H. F. Kabat (Eds.), *Chronobiology: 1982–1983.* Basel: S. Karger, pp. 345–349.
   A thorough discussion of the research on sleep disorders in the older adult.

REFERENCES

Beck, A. T., Rush, A. J., Shaw, B. F., & Emery, G. (1979). *Cognitive therapy of depression.* Englewood Cliffs, NJ: Prentice-Hall.
Bootzin, R. R., & Engle-Friedman, M. (1987). Sleep disturbances. In L. L. Carstensen & B. A. Edelstein (Eds.), *Handbook of clinical gerontology.* New York: Pergamon Press, pp. 238–251.
Carlson, C. R., Ventrella, M. A., & Sturgis, E. T. (1987). Relaxation training through muscle stretching procedures: A pilot case. *Journal of Behavior Therapy and Experimental Psychiatry, 18,* 121–126.
Chambless, D. L., Goldstein, A. J., Gallagher, R., & Bright, P. (1986). Integrating behavior therapy and psychotherapy in the treatment of agoraphobia. *Psychotherapy, 23,* 150–159.
Davis, M., Eshelman, E. R., & McKay, M. (1982). *The relaxation and stress reduction workbook.* Oakland, CA: New Harbinger.
Friedman, M., & Rosenman, R. H. (1974). *Type A behavior and your heart.* New York: Alfred A. Knopf.
Goldfried, M. R., & Trier, C. S. (1974). Effectiveness of relaxation as an active coping skill. *Journal of Abnormal Psychology, 83,* 348–355.
Hoelscher, T. J., & Edinger, J. D. (1988). Treatment of sleep-maintenance insomnia in older adults: Sleep period reduction, sleep education, and modified stimulus control. *Psychology and Aging, 3,* 258–263.
Janis, I. L. (1983). The role of social support in adherence to stressful decisions. *American Psychologist, 38,* 143–159.
Knight, B. (1986). *Psychotherapy with older adults.* Beverly Hills, CA: Sage.
Lakein, A. (1973). *How to get control of your time and your life.* New York: Signet.
Lehrer, P. M. (1982). How to relax and how not to relax: A re-evaluation of the work of Edmund Jacobson. *Behaviour Research and Therapy, 20,* 417–428.
Lewinsohn, P. M., Munoz, R. F., Youngren, M. A., & Zeiss, A. M. (1986). *Control your depression.* Englewood Cliffs, NJ: Prentice-Hall.
Maddi, S. R., & Kobasa, S. C. (1984). *The hardy executive: Health under stress.* Homewood, IL: Dow Jones–Irvin.
Marlatt, G. A. (1985). Lifestyle modification. In G. A. Marlatt & J. R. Gordon (Eds.), *Relapse prevention.* New York: Guilford Press, pp. 280–348.

Martin, J. E., & Dubbert, P. M., (1987). Exercise promotion. In J. A. Blumenthal & D. C. McKee (Eds.), *Applications in behavioral medicine and health psychology: A clinician's source book.* Sarasota, FL: Professional Resource Exchange, pp. 361–398.

Prinz, P. N., & Raskind, M. (1978). Aging and sleep disorders. In R. L. Williams & I. Karacan (Eds.), *Sleep disorders: Diagnosis and treatment.* New York: John Wiley, pp. 303–321.

Rosenberg, R. S. (1984). Aging and biological rhythms: Complaints of insomnia in the elderly. In E. Haus & H. F. Kabat (Eds.), *Chronobiology: 1982–1983.* Basel: S. Karger, pp. 345–349.

Stuart, R. B. (1980). *Helping couples change: A social learning approach to marital therapy.* New York: Guilford Press.

Wolpe, J. (1969). *The practice of behavior therapy.* Oxford: Pergamon Press.

Worden, J. W. (1982). *Grief counseling and grief therapy.* New York: Springer.

Index

Abdominal breathing, 70; *see also* Breathing; Relaxation therapy
Activation, sleep drive/responsivity, 6–9
Age level; *see also* Elderly
   circadian rhythms and, 68–69
   delayed sleep phase syndrome and, 194
   pharmacotherapy and, 118, 120
   vicious circle model and, 167
Alcohol
   delayed sleep phase syndrome and, 200, 201
   pharmacotherapy and, 116
   sleep hygiene rules and, 68
   treatment selection strategy and, 140
Antidepressants; *see also* Depression; Pharmacology
   pharmacotherapy protocols and, 123–124
   sleep behavior management and, 181
Anxiety
   barriers to sleep and, 4
   early morning awakening insomnia, 209, 212
   elderly and, 239
   insomnia and, 156
   pharmacotherapy and, 119, 122–123
   predisposing factor, 11
   psychotherapy (short-term), 103, 112
   sleep behavior management, 176
   sleep restriction therapy, 61
   treatment selection strategy and, 137, 138, 140, 146–147
Arousal
   barriers to sleep and, 3

Arousal (*cont.*)
   functional chronic insomnia, 104, 106
   psychotherapy (short-term), 112
   stimulus control instructions and, 19
Associative control of sleep, 4–6
Asthma, 233
Autogenic training, 70; *see also* Relaxation therapy

Bed cue, stimulus control instructions, 19
Bedtime regularization, sleep hygiene rules, 68–69
Behavior therapy
   pharmacotherapy combined with, 117
   stimulus control (group setting), 32–34
   stimulus control instructions and, 21
Benzodiazepine sedative-hypnotics, 115; *see also* Pharmacology; Pharmacotherapy
Biofeedback, 70; *see also* Relaxation therapy
Body temperature rhythms
   sleep hygiene rules, 68
   wake-maintenance zone and, 9, 10
Breathing; *see also* Relaxation therapy
   abdominal breathing, 70
   good night's sleep model, 142
Bright light therapy
   body temperature rhythms and, 10
   delayed sleep phase syndrome and, 196, 199–200
   early morning awakening insomnia and, 207, 210–211, 214; *see also* Early morning awakening insomnia
   effectiveness discussed, 215–218

Caffeine
  pharmacotherapy and, 116
  psychotherapy and, 88
  sleep hygiene rules and, 68
Chronic illness, 223–236; see also Organic sleep pathology
  cardiogenic nocturnal dyspnea case study, 229–232
  hypnogenic dystonia case study, 228–229
  method of treatment, 224–228
  overview of, 223–224
  treatment applications, 232–234
Chronic insomnia: see Functional chronic insomnia
Chronicity, pharmacotherapy, 119
Chronic obstructive pulmonary disease (COPD)
  sleep disturbance and, 224
  treatment method and, 225
Chronic pain
  chronic illness and, 233–234
  treatment strategy and, 136–137
Circadian rhythm
  bright light therapy and, 210–211
  delayed sleep phase syndrome, 194, 198
  early morning awakening insomnia, 209–210
  good night's sleep model, 144
  sleep hygiene rules, 67–68
  sleep-wake schedule disorders, 191
  vicious circle model, 155
  wake-maintenance zone and, 10
Classical conditioning, associative control of sleep, 4–6
Clock, sleep hygiene rules, 67
Clonazepam, organic sleep pathology, 123; see also Pharmacotherapy
Coffee, sleep hygiene rules, 68; see also Caffeine
Cognitive relaxation, sleep behavior management, 179–180
Cognitive restructuring
  elderly and, 239
  good night's sleep model, 142–143
  sleep behavior management and, 178
Cognitive therapy
  combined therapy, 71–74
  psychotherapy (short-term), 103
Combined therapies
  pharmacotherapy/behavior therapy, 117

Combined therapies (cont.)
  sleep hygiene/relaxation therapy/cognitive strategies
    case history (successful), 74–79
    case history (unsuccessful), 79–82
    cognitive component, 71–74
    relaxation therapy component, 70–71
    sleep hygiene component, 65–70
Compliance: see Patient compliance
Conditioned insomnia, psychotherapy, 90
Conditioning, associative control of sleep, 4–6
Control needs, treatment selection strategy, 138, 145–146
Coping, functional chronic insomnia, 104
Core temperature: see Body temperature rhythms
Countertransference, psychotherapy, 95

Daily sleep log: see Sleep log
Deep breathing exercises: see Breathing
Delayed sleep phase syndrome, 193–205
  background of, 193–196
  case study (successful), 200–202
  case study (unsuccessful), 202–204
  method of treatment, 197–200
  overview of, 193
Depression
  barriers to sleep and, 3
  delayed sleep phase syndrome, 193, 195, 201
  early morning awakening insomnia, 212
  elderly and, 239
  insomnia and, 30, 156
  pharmacotherapy and, 115, 123–124
  predisposing factor, 11
  psychotherapy and, 89
  sleep behavior management, 176
  stimulus control instructions and, 23–24, 25
  treatment selection strategy and, 138
Disease-related insomnia: see Chronic illness; Organic sleep pathology
Dreaming, early morning insomnia, 209; see also Night terror
Drug abuse, delayed sleep phase syndrome, 200, 201; see also Alcohol; Substance abuse
Drug treatment: see Pharmacology
Dysthymia
  sleep behavior management and, 181

INDEX

Dysthymia (*cont.*)
  stimulus control instructions and, 25

Early morning insomnia, 207–220
  bright light and the sleep–wake cycle, 210–211
  case history in, 212–215
  differential diagnosis of, 208–210
  effectiveness discussed, 215–218
  overview of, 207–208
  symptoms of, 208
  treatment summarized, 218–219
Education (of patient)
  sleep behavior management, 175; *see also* Sleep behavior management
  treatment selection strategy, 139–140
Ego-supportive psychotherapy, described, 93–94
Elderly, 237–247; *see also* Age level
  case example (successful), 240–242
  case example (unsuccessful), 243–245
  circadian rhythms and, 68–69
  method of treatment, 238–249
  overview of sleep in, 237–238
  sleep drive and, 8
  sleep restriction therapy and, 51, 54
  stimulus control (group setting), 43–44
Electromyography, relaxation therapy, 71
Emotional arousal: *see* Arousal
Exercise
  delayed sleep phase syndrome, 195–196
  good night's sleep model, 142
  sleep hygiene rules, 67–68

Family counseling, described, 97
Family therapy, psychotherapy (short-term), 103
Flurazepam, sleep behavior management, 183–186
Forbidden zone: *see* Wake-maintenance zone
Functional chronic insomnia; *see also* Insomnia
  pharmacotherapy and, 115, 116
  psychotherapy (short-term), 104

Gestalt therapy, described, 95–96
Good night's sleep model; *see also* Treatment selection strategy
  attributes of, 134–135
  described, 141–145

Group psychotherapy, described, 97
Group stimulus control, 29–47; *see also* Stimulus control (group setting)

Hand temperature, relaxation therapy, 71
Hunger, sleep hygiene rules, 69
Hypnotics: *see* Pharmacology; Pharmacotherapy

Iatrogenic insomnia, 223
Insomnia; *see also* Functional chronic insomnia; Sleep
  barriers to sleep and, 2–4
  chronic illness and, 223–236; *see also* Chronic illness
  elderly and, 237–238
  functional chronic insomnia, 104
  overview of, 1–2
  predisposing, precipitating, and perpetuating factors in, 11–13
  sources of, 30, 156
  treatment revolution for, vii
  treatment variety for, viii

Life-style
  elderly and, 239
  treatment selection strategy and, 138
Light therapy: *see* Bright light therapy

Marriage counseling, described, 97
Meals, sleep hygiene rules, 69
Medical problems, treatment selection strategy, 136–137; *see also* Organic sleep pathology
Meditation
  relaxation therapy and, 70; *see also* Relaxation therapy
  sleep behavior management and, 179–180

Napping, sleep hygiene rules, 69
Neurosis, functional chronic insomnia, 104
Nicotine
  sleep hygiene rules, 68
  treatment selection strategy, 140
Night terror
  early morning awakening insomnia, 209
  vicious circle model and, 164
Nonrestorative sleep syndrome, pharmacotherapy, 115

Older adults: *see* Elderly

Organic sleep pathology, 30; *see also* Chronic illness
  assessment and, 31
  chronic illness and, 228
  pharmacotherapy protocols for, 122–123
  psychotherapy and, 89
  psychotherapy (short-term) and, 105
  sleep restriction therapy contraindicated, 51–52
  treatment selection strategy and, 137
Outcomes
  chronic illness and, 228–232
  combined therapy (sleep hygiene/relaxation therapy/cognitive strategies), 74–82
  delayed sleep phase syndrome, 200–204
  early morning awakening insomnia, 212–218
  elderly and, 240–245
  pharmacotherapy, 124–126
  psychotherapy, 94, 100
  psychotherapy (short-term), 106–111
  sleep restriction therapy, 60–62
  stimulus control (group setting), 41–42
  treatment selection strategy, 145–149
  vicious circle model, 161–170

Pain
  chronic illness and, 233–234
  treatment strategy and, 136–137
Patient compliance, sleep restriction therapy, 52, 53
Pharmacology, 85–86
  associative control of sleep and, 5–6
  chronic illness and, 225–228, 232–233, 233–234
  early morning insomnia, 212
  sleep behavior management and, 181, 183–186
  sleep drive and, 8
  sleep hygiene rules and, 69–70
  stimulus control (group setting), 44
  treatment selection strategy, 137, 140
  withdrawal of hypnotics, stimulus control instructions, 20–21, 24
Pharmacotherapy, 115–129
  behavior treatment combined with, 117
  case histories in, 124–126
  contraindications for, 127
  delayed sleep phase syndrome, 196, 200
  discontinuation of medication, 126–127

Pharmacotherapy (*cont.*)
  indications for, 115–117
  medication choice, 117–120
    dosages, 120
    duration of effect, 118–119
    metabolism type, 120
    onset of effect, 119–120
  method of treatment, 120–124
    antidepressant use, 123–124
    general rules, 120–122
    protocol examples for specific diagnoses, 122–123
  overview of, 115
  side effects, 127
  sleep behavior management and, 178
  vicious circle model, 159–160
Polysomnography
  delayed sleep phase syndrome, 197, 198, 201–202, 203
  early morning awakening insomnia, 213
  organic sleep pathology and, 31
  pharmacotherapy and, 116
  psychotherapy (short-term) and, 105
  sleep behavior management, 176
Problem diary, good night's sleep model, 143
Progressive muscle relaxation; *see also* Relaxation therapy
Psychoanalysis, described, 92–93
Psychoanalytic psychotherapy, described, 93
Psychopathology
  barriers to sleep, 3–4
  delayed sleep phase syndrome, 195
  early morning awakening insomnia, 208
  elderly, 239
  Gestalt therapy, 96
  insomnia, 30
  psychotherapy, 90, 94–95
  psychotherapy (short-term), 105, 112
  sleep behavior management, 176
  stimulus control instructions, 25–26
  treatment selection strategy, 137
Psychotherapy (general), 85–86, 87–101
  case history, 98–100
  classical psychoanalysis, 92–93
  differential diagnosis, 88–89
  ego-supportive psychotherapy, 93–94
  Gestalt therapy, 95–96
  group psychotherapy, 97
  indications for, 90

INDEX

Psychotherapy (general) (*cont.*)
  marriage and family counseling, 97
  outcomes, 94
  overview of, 87–88
  psychoanalytic psychotherapy, 93
  referral considerations, 90–92
  sleep behavior management, 182
  time-limited, dynamic psychotherapy, 94–95; *see also* Psychotherapy (short-term)
  vicious circle model, 159, 160, 170–171
Psychotherapy (short-term), 103–114
  case example (successful), 106–109
  case example (unsuccessful), 109–111
  discussion of, 111–113
  functional chronic insomnia and, 104–105
  method of, 105–106
  overview of, 103–104

Rapid-eye-movement (REM) sleep, psychotherapy, 89
Relaxation therapy
  combined therapy, 70–71
  elderly and, 239
  good night's sleep model, 142
  sleep behavior management and, 179–180
  vicious circle model, 160, 171
Resistance, psychoanalysis, 92
Responsivity, activation/sleep drive, 6–9
Restless legs syndrome: *see* Organic sleep pathology
Ritual, good night's sleep model, 141–142

Schizophrenia, insomnia, 30
Secondary gains, treatment selection strategy, 138
Self-reports; *see also* Daily sleep log
  delayed sleep phase syndrome, 198–199
  pharmacotherapy and, 119
  sleep behavior management, 177
  treatment selection strategy and, 135–136
Short-term insomnia, pharmacotherapy protocols for, 122
Short-term psychotherapy: *see* Psychotherapy (short-term)
Sleep
  associative control of, 4–6
  barriers to, 2–4

Sleep (*cont.*)
  perception of, 10–11
  timing of, 9–10
Sleep apnea, 229–232
Sleep behavior management, 175–189
  case study (successful), 180–183
  case study (unsuccessful), 183–188
  implementation of, 177–180
  overview of, 175
  patient selection and management in, 176
  treatment scheme, 176–177
Sleep deprivation therapy: *see* Sleep restriction therapy
Sleep diary: *see* Sleep log
Sleep disturbance threshold, 7–9
Sleep drive, activation/responsivity, 6–9
Sleep history questionnaire, 30
Sleep hygiene
  combined therapy, 65–70
  elderly and, 239
  sleep behavior management and, 177–178
Sleep hygiene rules
  listing of, 66–70
  stimulus control (group setting), 34, 35
Sleep log
  cognitive strategies and, 71
  delayed sleep phase syndrome, 198–199
  good night's sleep model, 143, 148
  sample of, 72, 73
  sleep behavior management, 177, 182
  sleep restriction therapy and, 51
  stimulus control (group setting), 31, 37
  stimulus control instructions, 20
  treatment selection strategy, 140
  vicious circle model and, 168
Sleep restriction therapy, 49–63
  assessment in, 50–51
  case examples, 53–60
  early morning insomnia, 214
  method of, 51–53
  outcomes, 60–62
  overview of, 49
  psychotherapy (short-term), 103
  sleep drive and, 6–7
  treatment selection strategy, 140
Sleep-wake schedule disorders
  delayed sleep phase syndrome, 193–205; *see also* Delayed sleep phase syndrome

Sleep-wake schedule disorders (*cont.*)
  early morning awakening insomnia, 207–220; *see also* Early morning awakening insomnia
  overview of, 191
Snacks, sleep hygiene rules, 69
Socioeconomic class, stimulus control (group setting), 44
Stimulants, sleep drive and, 8; *see also* Caffeine; Pharmacology
Stimulus control (group setting), 29–47
  method of study, 30–34
    assessment, 30–32
    behavior therapy elements, 32–34
  older adults, 43–44
  overview of, 29–30
  predictors of outcomes, 41–42
  sleep maintenance clients, 42–43
  treatment sessions in, 34–41
Stimulus control (individual), 19–28
  case history (successful), 23–25
  case history (unsuccessful), 25–27
  elderly and, 239
  good night's sleep model, 141
  intake method for study, 20–21
  listing of, 21–23
  overview of, 19–20
  psychotherapy (short-term), 103
Stress
  perpetuating factor, 12–13
  treatment selection strategy and, 136
  vicious circle model, 160
Substance abuse
  delayed sleep phase syndrome, 200, 201
  pharmacotherapy contraindication, 127

Thought stopping, good night's sleep model, 143
Time in bed, curtailment of, sleep hygiene rules, 66
Time-limited, dynamic psychotherapy, described, 94–95; *see also* Psychotherapy (short-term)
Tobacco: *see* Nicotine
Transference, 92–93, 95
Treatment selection strategy, 133–153
  assessment in, 135–139
  case study (successful), 145–147
  case study (unsuccessful), 147–149
  overview of, 133–135
  treatment program, 139–145
    education, 139–140
    good night's sleep model, 141–145
    learning factors, 140
Tricyclic antidepressants, pharmacotherapy protocols, 123–124; *see also* Depression; Pharmacology
Trying to sleep, sleep hygiene rules, 67
Tryptophan, sleep hygiene rules, 69

Vicious circle model, 155–174
  background of, 156–157
  case example (successful), 161–167
  case example (unsuccessful), 167–170
  discussed, 170–172
  method of treatment, 157–161
  overview of, 155–156

Wake-maintenance zone, timing of sleep, 9–10